IMMUNOLOGY AND IMMUNE SYSTEM DISORDERS

AUTOANTIBODIES

DETECTION, PATHOGENICITY AND HEALTH IMPLICATIONS

IMMUNOLOGY AND IMMUNE SYSTEM DISORDERS

Additional books in this series can be found on Nova's website under the Series tab.

Additional e-books in this series can be found on Nova's website under the e-books tab.

PUBLIC HEALTH IN THE 21ST CENTURY

Additional books in this series can be found on Nova's website under the Series tab.

Additional e-books in this series can be found on Nova's website under the e-books tab.

IMMUNOLOGY AND IMMUNE SYSTEM DISORDERS

AUTOANTIBODIES

DETECTION, PATHOGENICITY AND HEALTH IMPLICATIONS

GRAHAM E. JENKINS
AND
JOANNE I. HALL
EDITORS

Nova Science Publishers, Inc.
New York

For permission to use material from this book please contact us:
Telephone 631-231-7269; Fax 631-231-8175
Web Site: http://www.novapublishers.com

NOTICE TO THE READER

Additional color graphics may be available in the e-book version of this book.

LIBRARY OF CONGRESS CATALOGING-IN-PUBLICATION DATA

ISBN: 978-1-62081-560-1
Library of Congress Control Number: 2012935164

Published by Nova Science Publishers, Inc. † New York

CONTENTS

PREFACE

Autoantibodies that are directed against self antigens are called autoantibodies. Not all autoantibodies are harmful. Autoantibodies can be useful in the removal of cell debris during inflammation. Some autoantibodies may be the actual pathogenic agents of autoimmune disease, the secondary consequences of tissue damage, or the harmless footprints of an etiologic agent. In this book, the authors present current research in the detection, pathogenicity and health implications of autoantibodies. Topics include the implicated autoantibodies in kidney disease and Alzheimer's disease; autoimmunity in cardiovascular disease; detection and analysis of natural autoantibodies; and B Cells and autoantibodies in multiple sclerosis.

Chapter I - Pathogenic IgG autoantibodies can be initiated in experimental animals following injections of certain tissue components in adjuvants. Eg. slowly progressive Heymann nephritis, an experimental autoimmune kidney disease, can be produced in a susceptible strain of rat by IP injections of a nephritogenic antigen (derived from the brush border region of the renal proximal convoluted tubules) in an adjuvant. The developing pathogenic IgG autoantibodies target primarily the brush border localized nephritogenic antigen causing an autoimmune kidney disease; and secondarily, the glomerular fixed nephritogenic antigen, resulting in a membranous glomerulonephritis. During the course of the disease, pathogenic IgG autoantibodies can be detected on renal biopsy specimens of rats with slowly progressive Heymann nephritis by the direct fluorescence antibody test staining the brush border zone of cells in a diffuse pattern and the glomeruli in a beaded pattern. These autoantibodies are also present in the circulation (with various antibody titres) and utilizing the indirect fluorescence antibody test, normal frozen rat kidney sections show staining of the brush border localized nephritogenic antigen. If the modified nephritogenic antigen is present continually in the system then it will maintain pathogenic IgG autoantibody production and in turn causes a chronic progressive kidney disease. Besides pathogenic IgG autoantibodies, non-pathogenic IgM autoantibodies – also directed against the nephritogenic antigen – are present in the circulation. Their role is to assist in the elimination of native and modified nephritogenic antigens from the circulation. Through this process, IgM autoantibodies minimize pathogenic IgG autoantibody mediated injuries. Utilizing the immune system's natural abilities – to terminate pathogenic autoimmune kidney disease causing IgG autoantibody production – the authors employed a new vaccination technique that the authors developed and call modified vaccination technique. The modified vaccination technique can increase the level of circulating non-pathogenic IgM autoantibodies – directed against the nephritogenic antigen – and able to terminate immunopathological processes, specifically and without side effects by assisting in the elimination of modified and native target antigens from the system. The modified vaccination technique was able to prevent and treat the autoimmune kidney disease slowly progressive Heymann nephritis in rats (terminating the ongoing immunopathological processes); and tolerance to the native nephritogenic antigen was regained. The health implications of the modified vaccination technique – by providing appropriate information to the cells of the immune system to respond with increased non-pathogenic IgM autoantibodies – promises to prevent/terminate autoimmune diseases of humans as well.

Chapter II - Complement is an essential humoral component of the innate immune system. It participates in various physiological processes including the destruction of pathogens, waste disposal, inflammation, modulation of the activation of innate and adaptive immune cells, and tissue regeneration. The complement system consists of more than forty soluble and membrane-bound proteins, which form three major activation pathways and a terminal complement pathway, regulate the system and mediate biological functions such as cell activation. Complement deficiencies and malfunctions are associated with various infectious, inflammatory and immune disorders. Dysregulation of the alternative complement pathway is involved in the pathogenesis of the kidney diseases atypical hemolytic uremic syndrome and dense deposit disease. Factor H is a major inhibitor of the alternative complement pathway. Certain factor H mutations and autoantibodies against this regulatory protein are associated with atypical hemolytic uremic syndrome and dense deposit disease. The anti-factor H autoantibody-associated forms of these diseases require a corresponding treatment. This review provides an overview of the main factor H functions and the role of anti-factor H autoantibodies in kidney diseases. Furthermore, the problems of anti-factor H autoantibody detection, studies on the functional relevance and potential pathogenicity of such autoantibodies, and the importance of prompt autoantibody detection for the selection of appropriate treatment for the affected patients are discussed.

Chapter III - Alzheimer's disease (AD), the most common form of dementia affecting elderly people, is characterized by progressive cognitive decline accompanied by functional impairment, spatiotemporal disorientation and behavioral disturbances. The main histopathological features of the disease include extracellular accumulation of β- amyloid plaques, formation of intracellular neurofibrillary tangles, synaptic loss and neuronal cell death. A growing body of evidence suggests that the "autoimmune hypothesis" may play a critical role to AD pathogenesis. Significant changes both on the number as well as the spectrum of autoantibodies have been observed in the serum and cerebrospinal fluid (CSF) of AD patients, as compared to healthy elderly people. Interestingly, the targets of AD-related autoantibodies are not only neuronal proteins but also non-neuronal antigens displaying various cellular activities. In this review the authors discuss the current knowledge on the nature and role of autoantibodies that have been implicated in the disease onset and/or progression. The authors further discuss the potential therapeutic approaches based on these findings.

Chapter IV - Autoimmunity is becoming a fairly common issue in healthcare with a clinical syndrome present in up to 8% of the US population. Of all autoimmune conditions, there are more than 80 subtypes that are caused by various autoantibodies against a somatic cell type or tissue. It is the prevailing hypothesis that conditions such as preeclampsia (PE) and cardiomyopathy are the direct cause of autoimmune antibodies directed to receptors within the body. For instance, agonistic autoantibodies activating the angiotensin-1 receptor (AT_1R) and implicated in hypertension, proteinuria, and inhibition of vascular growth. This activating autoantibody (AT_1-AA) plays an integral role in PE. Additionally, earlier studies have shown the role of autoantibodies directed against the β_1-adrenergic receptor (β_1R-AA) in dilated cardiomyopathy and hypertension. The overall impact to patients with autoantibody-induced illnesses can include significant morbidity, concurrent illnesses, or mortality. Overall, these studies implicate the pathophysiologic role of autoantibody in these diseases. Of significance, these findings reveal an earlier diagnostic possibility and autoantibody targeted therapies in the disease treatment.

Chapter V - A normal immune system contains autoantibodies against self-antigens, termed as termed natural autoantibodies (NAAbs). NAAbs are found in many species, and appear to be conserved through evolution. The physiological significance of NAAbs is not well understood; however, it is postulated that NAAbs have various biological roles, such as first line protection against infection, immunoregulation, and clearance of altered self antigens. Recently, the authors have detected NAAbs against insulin in healthy cats while developing an enzyme-linked immunosorbent assay (ELISA) for determining feline serum insulin concentration. The authors study showed that feline NAAbs against insulin were polyclonal/polyreactive and had a high affinity and binding capacity. In this review, the authors outline the nature of NAAbs and the methods for detecting and analyzing of NAAbs, including ELISA for screening, affinity chromatography, competitive radioimmunoassay, and epitope analysis.

Chapter VI - Antibodies that are directed against self antigens are called autoantibodies. Not all autoantibodies are harmful. Autoantibodies can be useful in the removal of cell debris during inflammation, and autoantibodies to inflammatory cytokines can protect against untoward inflammation. Some autoantibodies may be the actual pathogenetic agents of autoimmune disease, the secondary consequences of tissue damage, or the harmless footprints of an etiologic agent. They can also inform us about basic mechanisms of loss of tolerance and inflammation in patients with autoimmune diseases. Autoantibodies can be present before the onset of some autoimmune diseases, show remarkable specificity and serve as biomarkers providing an opportunity for diagnosis and therapeutic intervention. Titers of some autoantibodies are increased in infections and in a variety of autoimmune diseases and are of little help in the differential diagnosis of disease. By contrast, most of the autoantibodies found in systemic autoimmune diseases are not detected in chronic infections. A negative result for antinuclear antibody (ANA) makes the diagnosis of systemic lupus or other systemic autoimmune disease unlikely, whereas a positive test with a high titer strongly supports the diagnosis. Likewise, in contrast to the high sensitivity and low specificity of rheumatoid factors (RFs) for rheumatoid arthritis, the anti-CCP autoantibody generally has a sensitivity of approximately 50%, but the specificity might be as high as 98%. Approximately 90% of patients with undifferentiated arthritis and raised anti-CCP auto-antibody titers will develop rheumatoid arthritis within few years. The specificity of many auto-antibodies has great diagnostic utility and might also have predictive value, such as with anti-CCP autoantibodies in rheumatoid arthritis. The specificity of autoantibodies in systemic auto-immunity also suggests an intimate relationship with disease pathogenesis. Few autoantibodies can be used alone to diagnose an autoimmune disease, because individuals without overt clinical disease, particularly relatives of patients with autoimmune diseases, might have detectable titers. Furthermore, some autoantibodies, although highly specific, are present only in a minority of patients. For example, autoantibodies to Smith occur in <30% of patients with systemic lupus. For these reasons, detection of autoantibodies is usually used to confirm a clinical diagnosis or help to define a subset of patients within a diagnostic category. In this chapter the authors discuss, the roles played by autoantibodies in the etiology, pathogenesis and diagnosis of autoimmune diseases with reference to the authors own experience in this field.

Chapter VII - During the last decades, investigations into MS have centered predominantly on the pathogenic role of autoreactive T cells rather than B cells. Recently, more evidence for a role of the humoral immune response in the MS pathogenesis is provided by the efficiency of novel treatment strategies; the preliminary positive results of intravenous immunoglobulin (IVIG) and B cell targeting therapy (Rituximab) in a group of MS patients have led to a renewed focus on B cells and autoantibodies in this autoimmune disease. In this chapter, the authors describe the humoral immune response in MS. The B cell repertoire in healthy individuals and MS patients is discussed. Next, B cell functions in MS as well as B cell migration and survival in the central nervous system (CNS) are outlined. An overview is given of the evidence for the involvement of B cells in the pathogenesis of MS. Finally, different technologies for the study of the humoral reactivity profile in MS are described, including autoantibody profiling and B cell reactivity analysis. Phage display and B cell immortalization are described in more detail as examples of both reactivity screening approaches. The analysis of the reactivity profile of B cells and autoantibodies in MS is relevant for the identification of novel disease markers for diagnosis, prognosis and theranostics, as well as for the elucidation of the underlying disease processes to discover highly needed novel therapeutic targets for the disease. Multiple sclerosis (MS) has been regarded as a T cell mediated disorder for a long time. This focus on T cells was partly attributed to the long-standing observation that an important lymphocytic subset in MS lesions was composed of T cells. In addition, the clear pathogenic effect of myelin-reactive T cells in the animal model of MS, experimental autoimmune encephalomyelitis (EAE), contributed to the belief that autoreactive T cells were at the center of the MS pathogenic processes. Recent studies into B cell and antibody-depleting therapeutic strategies in MS have renewed interest into the involvement of B cells in the underlying disease pathogenesis. During the last decades, more and more evidence has been collected for an important role of the humoral immune response in MS pathogenesis. In this chapter, the B cell repertoire in healthy individuals and MS patients will first be discussed. Next, B cell functions in MS, B cell migration and survival in the central nervous system (CNS) are outlined. An overview is given of the evidence for the involvement of B cells in the pathogenesis of MS. Finally, different technologies for the study of the humoral reactivity profile in MS are described.

In: Autoantibodies
Editors: G. E. Jenkins and J. I. Hall

ISBN: 978-1-62081-560-1

Chapter I

IMPLICATED AUTOANTIBODIES IN A KIDNEY DISEASE

Arpad Zsigmond Barabas[1 1]***, Chad Douglas Cole***[2]***, Rene Lafreniere***[1] ***and Donald Mackay Weir***[3]

[1]Department of Surgery, University of Calgary, Calgary, Alberta, Canada
[2]Department of Neurosurgery, University of Utah, US
[3]University of Edinburgh Medical School, Edinburgh, Scotland

ABBREVIATIONS

aab, autoantibody; aag, autoantigen; ab, antibody; ag, antigen; BB, brush border; FCA, Freund's complete adjuvant; GBM, glomerular basement membrane; G/M, ratio between IgG/IgM; HN, Heymann nephritis; IC, immune complex; ICGN, immune complex glomerulonephritis; MGN, membranous glomerulonephritis; MVT, modified vaccination technique; MW, molecular weight; rKF3, rat kidney fraction 3; rarKF3, rat anti-rat kidney fraction 3; SPHN, slowly progressive Heymann nephritis

---

1 Corresponding author: University of Calgary, Department of Surgery, 2808 Health Sciences Centre, 3330 Hospital Dr. NW, Calgary, Alberta, Canada T2N 4N1 Tel: 403-220-8901, Fax: 403-270-8795, E-mail: *barabas@ucalgary.ca* (A. Z. Barabas).

ADDITIONAL WELL KNOWN ABBREVIATIONS

C3, C5b-9, IgG, IgM, IP, NK cells, T cells

ABSTRACT

Pathogenic IgG autoantibodies can be initiated in experimental animals following injections of certain tissue components in adjuvants. Eg. slowly progressive Heymann nephritis, an experimental autoimmune kidney disease, can be produced in a susceptible strain of rat by IP injections of a nephritogenic antigen (derived from the brush border region of the renal proximal convoluted tubules) in an adjuvant. The developing pathogenic IgG autoantibodies target primarily the brush border localized nephritogenic antigen causing an autoimmune kidney disease; and secondarily, the glomerular fixed nephritogenic antigen, resulting in a membranous glomerulonephritis.

During the course of the disease, pathogenic IgG autoantibodies can be detected on renal biopsy specimens of rats with slowly progressive Heymann nephritis by the direct fluorescence antibody test staining the brush border zone of cells in a diffuse pattern and the glomeruli in a beaded pattern. These autoantibodies are also present in the circulation (with various antibody titres) and utilizing the indirect fluorescence antibody test, normal frozen rat kidney sections show staining of the brush border localized nephritogenic antigen.

If the modified nephritogenic antigen is present continually in the system then it will maintain pathogenic IgG autoantibody production and in turn causes a chronic progressive kidney disease.

Besides pathogenic IgG autoantibodies, non-pathogenic IgM autoantibodies – also directed against the nephritogenic antigen – are present in the circulation. Their role is to assist in the elimination of native and modified nephritogenic antigens from the circulation. Through this process, IgM autoantibodies minimize pathogenic IgG autoantibody mediated injuries. Utilizing the immune system's natural abilities – to terminate pathogenic autoimmune kidney disease causing IgG autoantibody production – we employed a new vaccination technique that we developed and call modified vaccination technique. The modified vaccination technique can increase the level of circulating non-pathogenic IgM autoantibodies – directed against the nephritogenic antigen – and able to terminate immunopathological processes, specifically and without side effects by assisting in the elimination of modified and native target antigens from the system.

The modified vaccination technique was able to prevent and treat the autoimmune kidney disease slowly progressive Heymann nephritis in rats (terminating the ongoing immunopathological processes); and tolerance to the native nephritogenic antigen was regained. The health implications of the modified vaccination technique – by providing appropriate information to the cells of the immune system to respond with increased non-pathogenic IgM autoantibodies – promises to prevent/terminate autoimmune diseases of humans as well.

Keywords: Autoimmunity, Modified Vaccination Technique, Membranous Glomerulonephritis

INTRODUCTION

Autoimmune diseases occur "spontaneously" in approximately 5% of humans, in our population. Quite often the causal or initiating and maintaining agents are not known; though in recent years environmental, hormonal, geographic location etc. factors are implicated [1, 2, 6, 43, 53, 71, 77, 90, 91, 94, 95, 100, 107]. Perhaps environmental influences cause most of the autoimmune diseases in susceptible individuals by being in contact with such products as: alcohol, smoking, UV light, burns, drugs, chemicals, dyes, vaccines, trauma, infectious agents, toxins etc. that are able to chemically/structurally modify self antigens (ags) [23]. Quite often autoimmune diseases develop gradually in humans because most of the modifying agents are weak adjuvants, i.e., not powerful initiators of the disease. However, in certain experimentally induced autoimmune diseases in animals, the pathogenic immune response – against a target ag – can be accelerated, resulting in a rapidly progressive pathogenic immunological response against self. One of these rapidly progressive autoimmune diseases is Heymann nephritis (HN). It can be induced in susceptible strain of rats by multiple IP injections of a nephritogenic ag in Freund's complete adjuvant (FCA). Within eight weeks the developing autoimmune kidney disease is characterized by: high titred pathogenic IgG autoantibody (aab) response, targeting the brush border (BB) region of the renal proximal convoluted tubules and the glomerular localized nephritogenic ag, causing proteinuria and membranous glomerulonephritis (MGN) [14, 55, 56, 59]. Kidney biopsy specimens stained for rat IgG and complement components (C3, C5b-9) by the direct fluorescence antibody (ab) test have shown the glomerular capillary loops with a beaded pattern of fluorescence and the BB region of the renal proximal convoluted tubules with a diffuse staining pattern [14]. The developing IgG aabs were highly pathogenic and caused irreversibly progressive immune complex glomerulonephritis (ICGN). Even though most autoimmune diseases are slowly progressive in humans [6] (because weak adjuvants modify self ags mainly and patients often receive treatment as well) the long-term effects of immunological insults against a target ag can lead to functional and morphological changes in an organ by the developing pathogenic IgG aabs eg. in lupus, MGN. During the progressive phase of the autoimmune disease HN we have noticed that rats had not only high pathogenic IgG aab but also high non-pathogenic IgM aab [14] titred responses against the nephritogenic ag. The IgM aabs being cross-reactive are able to remove the modified and released native autoantigens (aags) from the circulation [23], thereby minimizing damage to the target organ. We have noticed during the course of our experiment (and others as well) that the pathogenic IgG aabs attack one or multiple aags (eg. in HN, the nephritogenic ag in the BB and the glomeruli) within an organ (attempting to remove/eliminate the target ags). If the immunopathological events proceed long enough they can cause irreversible damage, often leading to organ failure. We have also observed that parallel with the pathogenic IgG aab response the specific non-pathogenic IgM aab response (which is always present with a low ab titre in the circulation) is also detectable with an elevated ab titre [14, 15].

In this review article we describe how a slowly progressive experimental autoimmune disease, slowly progressive Heymann nephritis (SPHN) in rats is induced and maintained in its progression by pathogenic IgG aabs targeting the nephritogenic ag in the kidney [14]. We also describe how pathogenic immune responses can be down regulated by IgM aabs directed against the native nephritogenic ag [10, 15, 17, 26].

AUTOIMMUNITY

Generally speaking when autoimmunity is mentioned in the medical literature, a harmful or pathogenic immune response against self by cellular or humoral events is understood. It conjures in the mind of the reader a pathogenic immune response against a target ag within tissues, organs etc. often causing a chronic progressive autoimmune disease. However, as we have described and categorized autoimmunity in recent years, the term 'autoimmunity' encompasses four possible immune responses against self [8, 9, 12, 13]: two beneficial and two harmful ones.

One of the beneficial aspects of autoimmunity works through specific IgM aabs against intracytoplasmic ags [103], which are released into the circulation from damaged or end-of-life span cells. Specific IgM aabs assist in the removal [7, 98-100, 103] and eventual degradation of these large molecular weight (MW) components, into reusable small MW peptides in mononuclear cells [64, 69, 82, 104]. Specific IgM aabs are present in the circulation, usually with a low ab titre against intracytoplasmic components, throughout life [103]. In a physiological sense we are not tolerant to intracytoplasmic large MW components [101, 102]. IgM aabs are cross-reactive and able to react with native and modified native aags [23]. This property of the IgM aab is beneficial because by being able to remove eg. chemically or otherwise modified native aags from the system, it contributes to the prevention of autoimmune diseases [10, 15]. Through these processes tolerance to self is maintained. Essentially, these specific IgM aabs by assisting in the clearance of released intracytoplasmic ags prevent toxic accumulation and possible modifications of endogenous ags that could cause autoimmune diseases.

Another beneficial aspect of autoimmunity is manifested by the elimination of those emerging cells in the system which are cancerous, bearing cancer specific ags on their cell surfaces. If besides cell mediated immune responses by NK cells, humoral immune responses in the presence of complement are also able to play a part: lysing cancer cells, then elimination of such cells from the system is possible. Unfortunately, small MW cancer specific ags on cancer cell surfaces often do not evoke cytolytic immune responses [36, 63] and cancer will prevail [23]. In such instances therapeutic interventions are applied to control cancer growth/spread [33, 62, 85]. The targeted cancer cell released intracytoplasmic components (just like normal cell degradation products) are assisted in their removal by specific IgM aabs [49]. In rare cases, cancer specific ags, on cancer cell surfaces could get in a milieu where infectious agents derived chemical components could act as adjuvants. Under this condition a cancer specific ag plus an adjuvant could initiate a cancer cell killing lytic aab response. These pathogenic lytic IgG aabs in the presence of complement by lysing cancer cells could eliminate cancer. So far no bacterial, viral or toxic extracts have been found or produced for adjuvant application.

One of the harmful aspects of autoimmunity manifests in animals and humans in autoimmune diseases [44, 50, 96]. The medical community is most knowledgeable about this aspect of autoimmunity. However, scientists quite often use (in our view inappropriately) the term 'autoimmunity' to denote autoimmune disease related immune events, not considering the fact that it encompasses four aspects of immune responses against self [9]. From various experiments we have learnt how autoimmune diseases can be initiated and maintained in experimental animals by injecting purified tissue ags in adjuvants. Eg. to initiate HN – an experimental autoimmune kidney disease – HN nephritogenic ag [50, 57] is injected several times in FCA into rats to cause the disease. The injected modified ag evokes a pathogenic IgG aab response against the nephritogenic ag and causes an autoimmune disease targeting the BB localized nephritogenic ag of the renal proximal convoluted tubules and the glomerular localized HN ag resulting in MGN [50, 59, 60]. The aim of the developing IgG aabs is to damage and eliminate the BB associated nephritogenic ag from the system. If the rapidly progressive immunological insults are maintained then injuries to the BB and the glomeruli of the kidney will result in an irreversible kidney damage that will lead to renal failure and eventually to death. Parallel with the pathogenic IgG aab response non-pathogenic IgM aabs are also produced against the target nephritogenic ag [14]. The function of the IgM aab is to remove the modified and native nephritogenic ags from the circulation [64, 69, 76, 82, 89, 104] thereby lessening pathogenic IgG aab production by the pathogenic IgG aab producing cell lines, i.e., they need constant stimuli by the modified nephritogenic ag and/or by immune complexes (ICs) made up of various combinations of the nephritogenic ag and pathogenic aabs against them [14, 17, 20, 25]. Sufficient levels of protective specific IgM aabs, directed against the nephritogenic ag, could downregulate immunopathological processes [10, 15]. However, even if autoimmune disease causing processes come to a halt, memory for the autoimmune disease initiating/causing (ag or ag plus adjuvant) antigenic information are retained [75].

Another harmful aspect of autoimmunity manifests in the lack of pathogenic lytic IgG aab response against emerging cancer cells with well-defined cancer specific ags. This pathogenic IgG aab response would be the only beneficial response against a self related endogenous ag (and not pathogenic IgG aab responses against normal self ags as they occur in autoimmune diseases). However, we do not know how many times cancer cells emerge and are eliminated by anti-cancer cell immune mediated responses by NK and T cells [66], lytic IgG aabs etc. When cancer cells establish themselves in an organ and in secondary sites, often weak or ineffective immune responses are mounted only by the host and treatment is required by immunosuppressive agents, cytotoxic drugs etc. to prevent out-of-control multiplication of cancer cells. Cancer cells coming to the end of their life span or damaged/killed by the administered drug(s) release their intracytoplasmic ags into the surrounding areas. These large MW ags are assisted in their removal by non-pathogenic IgM aabs prior to being degraded into small MW peptides in mononuclear cells, just like any intracytoplasmic ags released from normal cells. This is a beneficial aspect of autoimmunity, i.e., clearance and re-utilization of damaged cellular products, but unfortunately it does not promote live cancer cell kill.

DETECTION OF AABS IN THE CIRCULATION AND *IN SITU* PATHOGENIC AAB RESPONSE AGAINST TARGET ANTIGENIC SITES IN THE KIDNEYS OF SPHN RATS

Our findings are illustrated in an experimental autoimmune kidney disease called SPHN [14, 16]. SPHN is a variant of HN. It can be induced by injections of a chemically modified HN ag or by HN ag in Alum [16, 17, 100] in a susceptible strain of rat. The developing autoimmune kidney disease is slowly progressive (like most human autoimmune diseases [46]) and there is time to investigate immunopathological processes/lesion developments leading to the autoimmune disease and MGN.

Serum samples obtained from individual rats with SPHN were analyzed by the indirect fluorescence ab tests as follows: dilutions of serum samples were incubated at RT° on 4μ thick sections of normal rat kidneys for 30 minutes; thereafter sections were washed in physiological saline and stained for 30 minutes for the presence of rat IgG and rat IgM aabs with appropriate dilutions of Alexa Fluor® 488 labelled goat anti-rat IgG (H + L) and goat anti-rat IgM abs (μ chain; Molecular Probes, Eugene, OR, US). Ab titres were expressed as reciprocals of the last dilutions of sera giving positive results [17]. Normal animal's sera had no pathogenic IgG aabs against normal rat kidney ags [14, 16]. However, a low ab titre against the BB region of the renal proximal convoluted tubules' BB was observed on the IgM ab stained sections [14, 16]. Repeated injections of the HN ag in Alum resulted in elevated IgG and IgM ab responses [14]. Sera from these rats showed typical staining of the BB region of the renal proximal convoluted tubules for rat IgG and IgM abs [14]. Those animals which were treated with ICs (containing [rat kidney fraction 3 (rKF3) ag X rat anti-rat kidney fraction 3 (rarKF3) ag IgM ab] rKF3) showed a range of ab responses against the BB region of the renal proximal convoluted tubules, but mainly low anti-pathogenic IgG aab titres [15, 17]. The G/M ratios in these animals were at or near zero [15]. Detailed description of the procedures and findings at various stages of SPHN in pre- and post-treated, post-treated and control untreated rats were documented [15].

Kidney sections of rats with SPHN, stained by the direct fluorescence ab test, showed typical diffuse beaded pattern of fluorescence for rat IgG, C3 and C5b-9 in the glomerular capillary loops [14]. Those rats' kidney sections which were obtained from pre-and post-treated rats with ICs ([rKF3 ag X rarKF3 ag IgM ab] rKF3) had smaller and fewer beaded deposits around the glomerular capillaries (these animals also had lower proteinurias compared to untreated controls with SPHN) [15]. Those animals' kidney sections which were obtained from control rats stained the BB region of the renal proximal convoluted tubules by the direct florescence ab test for rat IgG with a diffuse pattern; and with the beaded pattern the glomerulus, Bowman's capsule and the tubular basement membrane [14].

Pathogenicity of IgG aabs against Kidney Ags in SPHN

The pathogenicity of the developing aabs during the course of an experimental autoimmune kidney disease called SPHN will be discussed. Both HN and SPHN are excellent examples of an autoimmune disease. These experimental autoimmune diseases are initiated and maintained by pathogenic IgG aabs – following injections of a HN ag in adjuvants [14, 27, 40, 41, 50, 54, 57, 72, 73, 92, 95] – targeting the nephritogenic ag localized primarily in the BB, and in the glomeruli as well (other antigenic sites are targeted as well, where HN ag is temporarily trapped/present, i.e., in the mesangium, Bowman's capsule, tubular basement membrane, urine, circulation, at the site where HN ag was injected in adjuvants etc.) [14].

SPHN is similar in its development to human autoimmune diseases which also progress gradually. We shall describe those immunopathological events that are harmful and also those which are beneficial. Pathogenic IgG aabs are produced in rats following repeated injections of HN ag in Alum [14]. The maintenance of IgG aabs in the circulation requires constant or intermittent presence of chemically or otherwise modified HN ag [17, 75] (exacerbation). There are scientists who believe that once pathogenic IgG aabs are produced their continual production is maintained by long-lived plasma cells [37, 65, 106]. It seems that such events might take place by long-lived plasma cells; however, experimental findings support the necessity of the modified ag to be present in the system for pathogenic IgG aab response to continue [17, 75]. Once pathogenic IgG aabs are produced against the HN ag they target tissue localized/produced and circulating HN ags [11, 14, 17, 30, 68, 74, 88].

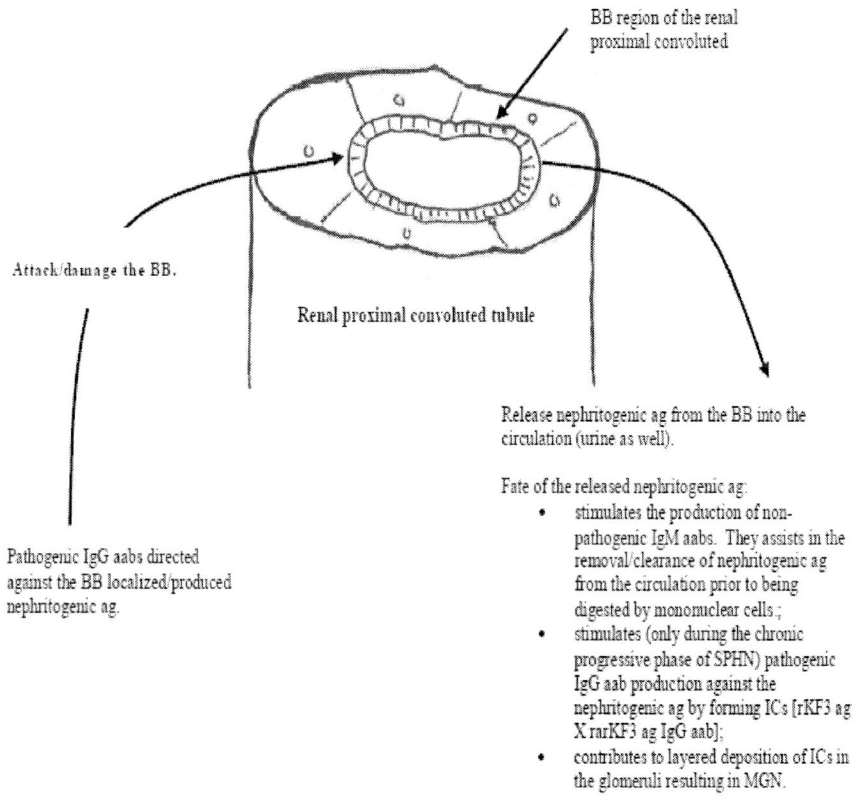

The primary target of the developing pathogenic rarKF3 ag IgG aab is the BB region of the renal proximal convoluted tubule. At this site the nephritogenic ag is produced and abundantly present. The developing pathogenic IgG aabs against the nephritogenic ag (produced following injections of the nephritogenic ag in adjuvant) attack/damage and release the nephritogenic ag from the BB zone of cells into the circulation.

Abbreviations: aab, autoantibody; ag, antigen; BB, brush border; IC, immune complex; MGN, membranous glomerulonephritis; rarKF3, rat anti-rat kidney fraction 3; rKF3, rat kidney fraction 3; SPHN, slowly progressive Heymann nephritis.

Figure 1. Autoimmune disease is due to pathogenic IgG aab response against the BB localized nephritogenic ag of the renal proximal convoluted tubule.

There are two main target sites where HN ag is present and attacked. The most abundant source of the HN ag is present in the BB region of the renal proximal convoluted tubules [95] where it is produced and fulfills an important role in the filtration of serum components. BB ags (including HN ag) even under normal physiological conditions shed frequently, releasing their ags into the circulation. This process is necessary for allowing the regenerated BB to function at a maximum efficiency.

Circulating pathogenic IgG aabs primarily target the BB region's cells causing damage [15] and release of the nephritogenic ag into the circulation. If the pathogenic IgG aab is present in the circulation for a prolonged period of time with a high ab titre then severe changes in the BB will occur and prevent its rapid regeneration and will contribute to non-selective proteinuria.

The pathogenic IgG aabs' primary target is the BB localized/produced nephritogenic ag causing a progressive autoimmune disease [Figure 1] (in another instance the target can be the glomerular localized neutral endopeptidase [86, 87]). As mentioned before, kidney sections of SPHN rats stain their BB region for rat IgG abs by the direct florescence ab test. The initial and subsequent production of the pathogenic IgG aab – directed against the nephritogenic ag – is achieved by the nephritogenic ag, introduced in an adjuvant to stimulate the cells of the immune system. Its continued production could also be maintained by injections of a chemically modified nephritogenic ag like azo-rKF3 ag [15, 17] and also by ICs that can be formed in the circulation such as [rKF3 ag X rat anti-azo rKF3 ag IgG aab] and [rKF3 ag X rarKF3 ag IgG aab] etc. Pathogenic IgG aabs targeting the BB are greatly responsible for the morphological and functional impairment of the affected kidneys.

It is noteworthy that native ags on their own do not initiate pathogenic IgG aab responses [16]. Native ags have to be modified chemically and/or structurally in order to obtain hapten-self protein conjugates [16]. These modified self proteins (not being quite self) are able to evoke pathogenic IgG aab responses [15, 17], essentially creating abs which are cross-reactive; being able to react with the ags that initiated their production (the hapten-self protein conjugates) and also with the native ags (the self proteins). In a roundabout way a pathogenic IgG aab response is initiated by the modified self ag; and if it is continuously present in the system then the pathogenic immune response is maintained, allowing the cross-reactive aab to cause damage in the target ag bearing organ [16].

The secondary target site – of the developing pathogenic IgG aab – resides in the glomeruli. There are two explanations how the nephritogenic ag becomes a target in the glomeruli and for the development of a MGN. The most accepted view is that the HN ag in the glomeruli is locally produced by the epithelial cells [58, 84]. It can be found intra-cellularly where it is associated with the endoplasmic reticulum, Golgi components and vesicular bodies. It is also present on epithelial cell surfaces and coated pits. It is believed that the HN ag is synthesized by the glomerular epithelial cells and transported to the epithelial cell membrane surfaces. To initiate reactivity with the HN ag the pathogenic IgG aab has to penetrate through the glomerular basement membrane (GBM) to meet up with the target ag, the epithelial cell localized/produced nephritogenic ag, and initiate the start and continuance of an ICGN in the presence of complement components (C3, C5b-9). Layered deposition of ICs (producing detectable ultra-structural changes especially in the GBM and epithelial cells) will follow as increased production of the nephritogenic ag by the epithelial cells and increased production of pathogenic IgG aabs against the nephritogenic ag becomes available. If this scenario is correct then treatment of SPHN and similar experimental and human autoimmune diseases, initiated by modified self ags, could only be treated by immunosuppressive agents, monoclonal abs etc. (to depress IgG aab production) and not by specific immune mediated interventions.

The second explanation for the development and enlargement of ICs on the epithelial side of the GBM is provided by the Barabas group. They observed that the glomeruli of normal rat kidneys contain small ICs composed of the nephritogenic ag and non-pathogenic IgM aabs directed against the nephritogenic ag [11] [Figure 2]. They also observed that those glomeruli – of newborn rats – which were not open to the circulation had no nephritogenic ags [34]; indicating that the nephritogenic ag was not produced by the epithelial cells but derived from a source other than the glomerular epithelial cells. The most logical possibility is that a certain portion of the BB released nephritogenic ag into the circulation [92, 93] penetrates through the GBM and joins with the circulation derived non-pathogenic rarKF3 ag IgM aabs and form ICs on the epithelial side of the GBM [11]. These small ICs do not cause morphologically discernible lesions in the glomeruli or proteinuria. When SPHN is induced in susceptible strain of rats by multiple injections of a nephritogenic ag in Alum, they start to produce cross-reactive pathogenic IgG aabs [14] that react with the modified and native nephritogenic ags. These aabs, getting through the GBM, join free antigenic sites of the HN ag on the epithelial side of the GBM and start the formation and continuation of layered deposition of ICs as shown on the diagrams [Figures 2 and 3].

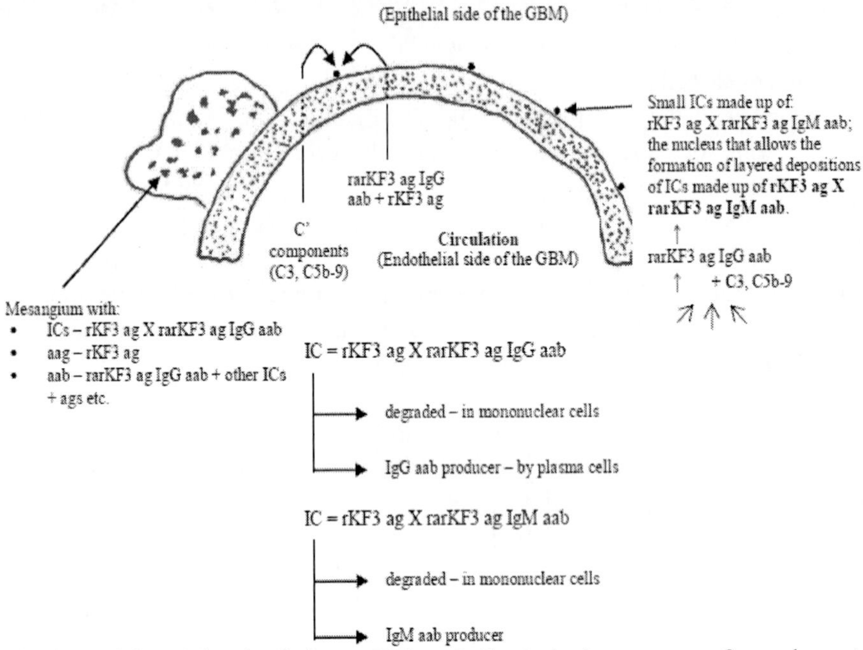

Initial reactivity of the circulating rarKF3 ag IgG aab, in the presence of complement, is with the free antigenic sites of the rKF3 ag which is present in the form of ICs [rKF3 ag X rarKF3 ag IgM aab] on the epithelial side of the GBM. Following the first step of reactivity, released nephritogenic ag from the BB region of cells (i.e., rKF3 ag) penetrating through the GBM joins free antigenic sites of the rarKF3 ag IgG aab, thus a layered deposition of ICs begins. The mesangium – to prevent obstructing glomerular filtration by large MW components – side lines and digests ags in its enzyme rich interior.

Abbreviations: aab, autoantibody; ag, antigen; C', complement components (C3, C5b-9); GBM, glomerular basement membrane; IC, immune complex; MW, molecular weight; rarKF3, rat anti-rat kidney fraction 3; rKF3, rat kidney fraction 3.

Figure 2**.** Secondary target of the developing pathogenic rarKF3 ag IgG aab is the glomerular localized (but not produced) nephritogenic ag.

Layered deposition of ICs on the epithelial side of the GBM by rarKF3 ag IgG aab with glomerular deposited nephritogenic ag in the presence of complement (C3, C5b-9) will continue; and cause additional abnormalities, i.e., fusion of epithelial cell foot processes over the deposits and projections/thickenings of the GBM in an attempt to surround and confine the ICs.These morphological abnormalities (together with damage to the BB) eventually lead to proteinuria [14, 15].

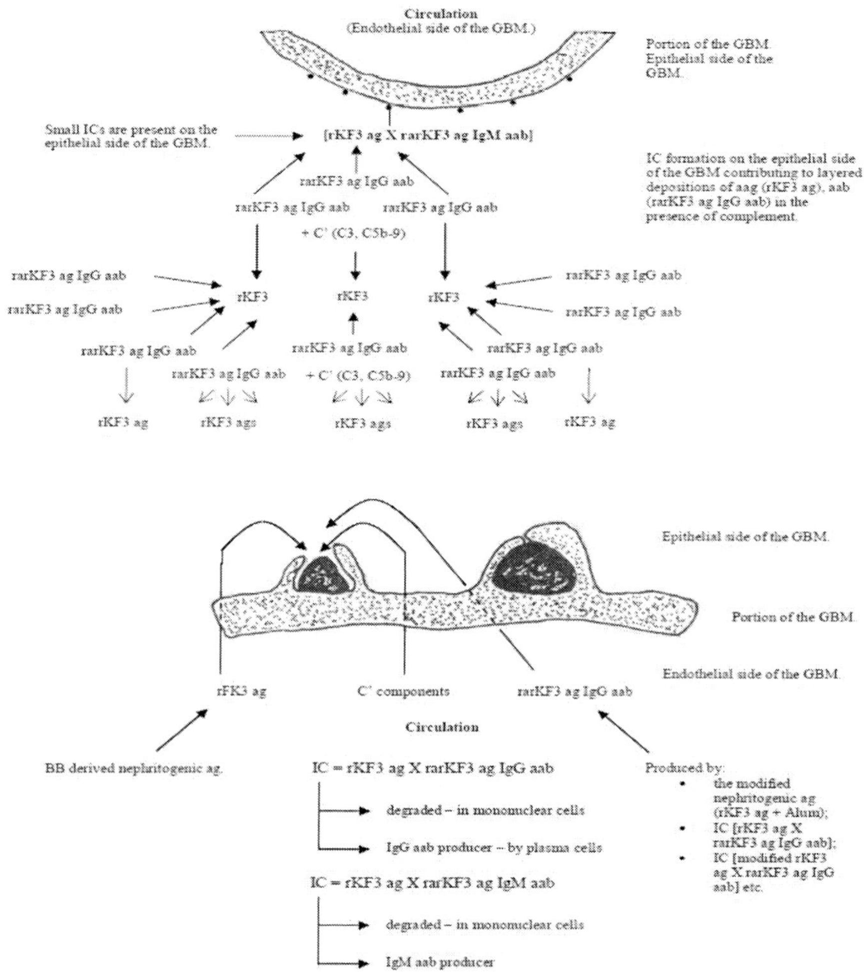

Continuous reactivity of circulating rarKF3 ag IgG aab, rKF3 ag and C' components on the epithelial side of the GBM produces large IC depositions that are partially or completely surrounded by basement membrane material. Morphological changes in the GBM and epithelial cells (fusion of foot processes) result in proteinuria. Immunological events lead to MGN.

Abbreviations: aab, autoantibody; ag, antigen; BB, brush border; C', complement components (C3, C5b-9); GBM, glomerular basement membrane; IC, immune complex; MGN, membranous glomerulonephritis; rarKF3, rat anti-rat kidney fraction 3; rKF3, rat kidney fraction 3

Figure 3. Enlargement of ICs on the epithelial side of the GBM by circulating aags (rKF3 ag) and aabs (rarKF3 ag IgG aab) in the presence of C'.

The glomerular lesion is not truly autoimmune in nature because the pathogenic IgG aab is not targeting a glomerular epithelial cell contained/produced nephritogenic ag. The glomerular lesion in the SPHN rat kidney is due to incidental immune events just as MGN is in humans. In our case it is due to the nature of the temporarily trapped BB derived nephritogenic ag in the form of immune complex (IC) [rKF3 ag X rarKF3 ag IgM aab] in the glomeruli [11] because of its physicochemical properties that allowed the formation of large ICs as depicted on Figure 3.

Non-Pathogenic IgM aabs against Kidney ags in SPHN

Specific non-pathogenic IgM aabs, directed against intracytoplasmic ags can be detected in the circulation throughout life [102]. In a physiological sense we are not tolerant to intracytoplasmic ags [101]. While intracytoplasmic ags are present within protective cell membranes they function without interference and fulfill their physiological roles. However, once they are released into the circulation they serve no further purpose.

When intracytoplasmic ags are released into the circulation from damaged or end of life span cells, specific IgM aabs assist in their removal [7, 98-100, 103] (to prevent their toxic accumulation or possible chemical/structural alterations to cause pathogenic aab induced autoimmune diseases) prior to being degraded by mononuclear cells [21, 29, 64, 76, 82, 104]. Generally speaking, in normal rats (and likely in humans as well) the IgM aab titre against intracytoplasmic ags is low [14]. However, if there is damage and release of massive amounts of intracytoplasmic components from cells into the circulation there is an immediate secondary ab response to produce increased production of intracytoplasmic ag clearing specific IgM aabs [17]. Such events are typically observed during a targeted attack, by pathogenic IgG aabs, against a special group of cells eg. as observed in SPHN and HN. Non-pathogenic IgM aabs are protective aabs. By efficiently clearing the system of released intracytoplasmic ags they are significant contributors for the maintenance of tolerance to self [Figure 4]. Specific IgM aab – during the development and progression of a pathogenic IgG aab driven autoimmune disease, as in SPHN – increases in ab titre against the target ag. The IgM aab is a cross-reactive ab. It is able to react with the ag that initiated its production, i.e., the modified ag, and native nephritogenic ag as well.

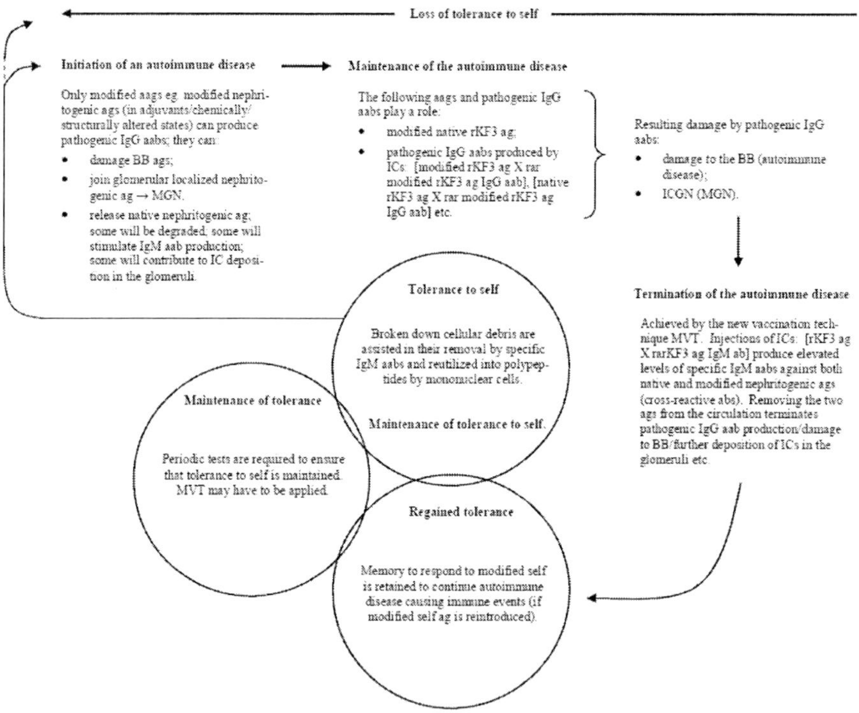

Only modified nephritogenic ags can produce pathogenic IgG aabs induced autoimmune diseases. The developing IgG aabs cause damage in the BB zone of cells of the renal proximal convoluted tubules (the autoimmune disease) and in the glomeruli by depositing ICs made up of the nephritogenic ags and pathogenic IgG aabs against them in the presence of complement (MGN). The MVT can prevent and when present terminate autoimmune disease causing events.

Abbreviations: aab, autoantibody; aag, aag; ag, antigen; BB, brush border; IC, immune complex; ICGN, immune complex glomerulonephritis; MGN, membranous glomerulonephritis; MVT, modified vaccination technique; rarKF3, rat anti-rat kidney fraction 3; rKF3, rat kidney fraction 3.

Figure 4. Initiation and maintenance of an autoimmune disease and regained tolerance to self by the MVT.

There are at least two instances when non-pathogenic IgM aabs could contribute to the development of an autoimmune disease. The first instance when a deficiently produced IgM aab [32] allows accumulation, stagnation and modification of a self ag by modifying agents (such as smoking, alcohol, chemicals, toxins, drugs etc.). In the second instance MGN can be established in HN susceptible strain of rats because ICs, [rKF3 ag X rarKF3 ag IgM aab], the nucleus for establishing MGN are present on the epithelial aspect of the

GBM [11] [Figure 3]. In spite of deficiencies the main role of the non-pathogenic IgM aab is to clear the system of liberated and modified intracytoplasmic ags. Even during an autoimmune disease it attempts to minimize damage by removing both modified and native aags which take part/contribute to disease development/maintenance. Through this process remission and even termination of an autoimmune disease causing event can be achieved.

HEALTH IMPLICATIONS

In a physiological sense we are not tolerant to our intracytoplasmic ags [101]. The presence of specific IgM aabs, throughout life, represents abs that are able to assist in the removal of native and modified native aags from the circulation [102] (secondary immune response). IgM aabs are clearing aabs of intracytoplasmic ags that are from time to time released from cells damaged by toxic agents or from cells coming to the end of their life spans [81, 98, 103]. IgM aabs are able to transfer ICs such as [native ag X autologous anti-native ag IgM aab], [modified native ag X autologous anti-modified native ag IgM aab] etc. into mononuclear cells, mesangial cells [11, 64, 76, 82] etc. for degradation into small MW peptides that can be re-utilized as new building blocks for functional or structural protein synthesis. The clearing function of these aabs is important because without their involvements, released native/modified aags could accumulate in the system and cause either toxic responses and/or pathogenic aab production that could lead to autoimmune diseases [16]. In our opinion specific IgM aabs significantly contribute to the maintenance of tolerance to self [Figure 4]. However, when the system is overwhelmed by massive release of intracytoplasmic ags – due to toxic damage to cells by agents such as chemicals, toxins, drugs, infectious agents etc. – the released ags could get modified, and the circulating IgM aabs will be unable to cope in the removal of cellular debris, and the likelihood of an autoimmune disease to develop is plausible [Figure 4]. IgM aabs through their physiological responses against self components fulfill one of the beneficial aspects of autoimmunity without which life as we know could not be sustained. Specific IgM aabs are cross-reactive. They are able to react with equal effectiveness, with both modified and native aags. For this reason IgM aabs are able to remove both aags from the system that could contribute to continuous pathogenic IgG aab production by stimulating the pathogenic IgG aab cell lines in various combinations, i.e., as a modified native ag alone;

modified native ag in the form of ICs [modified native ag X homologous anti-modified native ag IgG ab]; native ag (only during the chronic phase of the disease) in the form of ICs [native ag X homologous anti-native ag IgG ab] etc. By removing the pathogenic IgG aab producing and lesion contributing aags, specific IgM aabs slowdown immunopathological events and lead to remission and in certain instances termination of the autoimmune disease causing processes (regained tolerance to self) [Figure 4], without the use of drugs [10, 15, 17, 26]. It is wise not to target self ags with various harmful outside agents (i.e., smoking, alcohol, certain drugs, chemicals etc.) that could cause excessive damage to cells and modification of released intracytoplasmic ags that could lead to autoimmune diseases by pathogenic IgG aabs [1, 2, 71, 94]. Rather, assist the physiological role of the naturally occurring specific IgM aabs in the removal of intracytoplasmic ags to maintain tolerance to self by healthy lifestyles [47].

Another aab – which is present in the circulation only during the course of an autoimmune disease – is a pathogenic IgG aab. They are produced against certain self ags during the course of induction/progression of an autoimmune disease. Eg. in HN or SPHN pathogenic IgG aab response is evoked, following injections of a nephritogenic ag into rats in adjuvants [15, 17]. The developing pathogenic IgG aabs are directed against the target organ which contains the nephritogenic ag, i.e., the BB zone of cells of the renal proximal convoluted tubules and incidentally the epithelial aspect of the GBM as well [15]. Pathogenic rarKF3 ag IgG aabs targeting the BB zone of cells cause the autoimmune disease and reacting with the glomerular localized nephritogenic ag initiate/maintain MGN, as described earlier. As the disease progresses, animals will develop advanced morphological changes in the BB and glomeruli [15]. In the glomeruli layered depositions of ICs made up of the nephritogenic ag plus rat anti-rat nephritogenic ag IgG aab etc. in the presence of complement will initiate and maintain a rapidly progressive glomerulonephritis; and lesion development in the BB will be characterized by destroyed BB related zone of cells by the pathogenic IgG aab. The combined destructive lesions in the BB and in the glomeruli manifest in morphological and functional changes that result in non-selective proteinuria, defective retention/absorption of vitally important serum components etc. [15, 17]. Renal dysfunction will lead to weight loss, dehydration, protein loss, electrolyte imbalance etc. and in extreme cases, death.

Other health implicating factors in SPHN and similarly in humans with autoimmune diseases:

- in a pathological sense we are not tolerant to tissue components either if/when such ags are presented as modified self ags eg. hapten-self protein conjugates, self ags plus adjuvants etc. to the cells of the immune system. In such instances they will evoke a pathogenic IgG aab response against the target ag [3, 5, 48, 50, 95].;
- a pathogenic IgG aab initiated autoimmune disease (since the animal or human had no circulating pathogenic IgG aabs prior to disease) starts by a primary immune response; not by aabs against native ags but by aabs against chemically or structurally modified aags. The developing pathogenic IgG aabs are cross-reactive [50]. They are not only able to react with the modified native ags that initiated their production but also with native ags which are integral parts of an organ where they fulfill their functions. The production of the pathogenic IgG aab and its damaging effect will continue as long as the inciting agent – that is able to modify the self ag – is present in the system and produce cross-reactive pathogenic IgG aabs (secondary immune response) [17].;
- during continuous presence of a modifying agent in the system modified aags can be produced. Modified aags stimulate/maintain the pathogenic immune response (exacerbation) and the resulting pathogenic IgG aabs can cause significant damage to the target organ to such an extent that it could no longer contribute to good health [45, 50].;
- experiments carried out by us and others [17, 75] clearly revealed that not long-lived plasma cells [65, 83, 106] are responsible for the production of pathogenic IgG aabs but plasma cells that are programmed for pathogenic IgG aab production by the following ags and ICs (illustrated as they occur in SPHN) [Figure 3]: ags: rKF3 ag + FCA; chemically modified rKF3 ag (eg. azo-sonicated ultra-centrifuged rKF3 ag) etc.; ICs: [chemically modified rKF3 ag X rat anti-rat chemically modified rKF3 ag IgG aab]; [rKF3 ag X rat anti-rat chemically modified rKF3 ag IgG aab] etc. Note: rKF3 ag (released from the BB cells of the renal proximal convoluted tubules) can only take part in the maintenance (not in the initiation) of pathogenic IgG aab production during the chronic progressive phase of the autoimmune disease.;
- in the absence of modified and native nephritogenic ags in the circulation, autoimmune disease causing/contributing immune events come to a halt [17] (remission/termination), i.e., no further release of

nephritogenic ag from the BB by pathogenic rarKF3 ag IgG aabs that in turn could have contributed to additional pathogenic IgG aab production (by [rKF3 ag X rat anti-rat chemically modified rKF3 ag IgG aab]); no further deposition of ICs in the glomeruli; no stimulation of the pathogenic IgG aab cell lines by modified nephritogenic ag to produce pathogenic IgG aabs against the nephritogenic ag etc.;

- it is worthwhile to mention that during the course of an autoimmune disease, autoimmune disease causing events aim to eliminate the target ag from the system by the developing pathogenic IgG aabs. Such immune events can compromise and even terminate the normal functioning of an organ, as in SPHN causing renal failure [14].;
- there are autoimmune diseases which are slow to progress in certain individuals and only minimally present levels of circulating pathogenic IgG aabs indicate that pathogenic immune responses have begun without any clinical signs or symptoms [6]. The slow induction of the disease could be due to the presence of a mildly modifying agent in the system that modifies the pathogenic IgG aab inducing ag or efficient clearance of modified aag from the system by specific IgM aabs, or both.;
- G/M ratios that we have obtained in some of our SPHN experiments have shown that they can rapidly increase (due to IgG aab response) following re-stimulation [15, 17] of rats with the modified nephritogenic ag. The G/M ratio is a good indicator whether disease causing events are in decline (remission) or accelerated in favour of pathogenic IgG aab response (exacerbation). Only when the G/M ratio equals zero can we be certain that the autoimmune disease is in a state of dormancy [17].;
- immunological memory. Even if an autoimmune disease causing event appears to be terminated (i.e., G/M ratio is zero) the re-administration of the same modified native-like ag – that initiated the disease eg. in SPHN, rat azo-sonicated ultra-centrifuged rKF3 ag – will immediately bring about a pathogenic IgG aab response [17, 75] (secondary immune response) against the target nephritogenic ag in the BB region of the renal proximal convoluted tubule. For this, and other reasons as well, patients with pathogenic IgG aab induced autoimmune diseases should be regularly checked for the presence of both pathogenic and non-pathogenic aabs in the circulation [28, 52, 67, 78] [Figure 4].;

- presently, autoimmune diseases are treated with immunosuppressive agents. Though a pathogenic IgG aab response can be somewhat depressed by these drugs, the side effects they cause are numerous, of which infectious disease caused complications are the worst. The reason why immunosuppressive agents are not as beneficial as they are expected to be is due to the fact that a secondary immune response (like the one observed during the progressive phase of an autoimmune disease, where constant stimulation of immunological cell lines by a modified self ag maintains the pathogenic IgG aab production) cannot be as efficiently suppressed as a primary immune response initiated immune event.;

Prevention and Treatment of a Pathogenic IgG Aab Initiated and Maintained Experimental Autoimmune Disease by the Modified Vaccination Technique (MVT)

Treatment of autoimmune diseases is undertaken by immunosuppressive agents [28, 52, 67, 79]. Besides the many undesirable side effects they cause, they are unable to terminate autoimmune diseases specifically [52, 79]. It is long believed that effective immunotherapeutic solutions should be applied. The application of monoclonal abs [4, 31, 33, 37, 61, 80] in recent years has provided an alternate solution; but they are also non-specific in their actions and cause side effects [33]. The best solution would be to eliminate from the system those ags that are responsible for the pathogenic IgG aab production and lesion development [42]. As mentioned before pathogenic immune responses are initiated not by ags that are native ones but by those which are native-like, i.e., chemically or structurally modified native ags *per se* or native ags introduced with adjuvants or by ags showing molecular similarities to self ags [35, 38, 39, 70, 105] (molecular mimicry) etc. Self ags on their own do not initiate autoimmune diseases [14, 15, 17]. Furthermore, continuous production of IgG aabs is mainly maintained by modified aags [16, 17], though during the chronic phase of the disease native ags can also play a role, as we have described earlier. We also mentioned that specific IgM aabs are able to clear the system from released intracytoplasmic ags prior to being digested in mononuclear cells into small MW peptides. Since the nephritogenic ag is an intracytoplasmic ag – produced by the BB cells of the renal proximal convoluted tubules –it, and also the modified nephritogenic ag (since the IgM aab is a cross-reactive ab) should be removable from the circulation by specific IgM aabs in order to prevent/terminate:

- The nephritogenic ag to stimulate continuous IgG aab production by plasma cells; and
- The nephritogenic ag and the pathogenic IgG aab against it to cause chronic progressive ICGN.;

The vaccination technique that we have described and applied in several experiments is called MVT [8, 9, 12, 13, 18, 19, 22]. The MVT is able by ab information transfer to induce the production of the same ab with the same specificity against the target ag that is present in the inoculum, in the case of SPHN rarKF3 ag IgM aabs. The vaccine is made up of ICs [rKF3 ag X rarKF3 ag IgM ab] rKF3. The ICs are injected at frequent intervals to maintain an elevated IgM aab response to bring down pathogenic IgG aab production, i.e., in the absence of modified and native aags and ICs [modified rKF3 ag X rat anti-rat modified rKF3 ag IgG aab], [rKF3 ag X rat anti-rat modified rKF3 ag IgG aab] etc. in the circulation the pathogenic aab producing cell lines are no longer stimulated to produce autoimmune disease-causing pathogenic IgG aabs [23, 24].

The vaccination technique we have described is applicable for both prevention and treatment (termination) of a pathogenic IgG aab initiated and maintained autoimmune disease [8, 9, 18, 26], like that of SPHN (it should be applicable in exogenous ag initiated diseases as well [22]) [Table 1]. The vaccine is specific in its action; it stimulates exclusively the production of naturally occurring IgM aabs against the native target ag. The MVT assists the natural abilities of the immune system, by providing appropriate information, to initiate a corrective immune response through which the animals'/patients' disease causing immune events can be terminated and tolerance to the native self ag regained [Figure 4]. The MVT provides ag specific downregulation of pathogenic autoimmune responses directed against self components: in our case, down regulation of pathogenic IgG aab induced/maintained immune response against the BB associated nephritogenic ag. Downregulation/termination of the autoimmune disease is achieved without affecting any of the beneficial functions of the immune system; in other words, it is achieved specifically and without side effects.

CONCLUSION

The question is: are all the abs beneficial in a living systems' circulation? The answer simply is that not all of them are beneficial. There are those which result from inappropriately presented ags to the cells of the immune system. Since we are dealing with autoimmune disease related issues, we have concentrated on immune responses that are both beneficial and harmful to the host.

We already made the statement that in a physiological sense we are not tolerant to our intracytoplasmic ags throughout life. Since these ags are present within the internal environments of cells, and well protected by cell membranes, no immune response can be initiated against them. However, if cells are damaged by agents that are toxic [14, 81, 97-99] (such as hypoxia, certain drugs, chemicals, trauma, cold, pathogenic IgG aabs etc.) or as a consequence of coming to the end of their life spans, cell membranes rupture and intracytoplasmic components are released for recognition.

The fate of the released intracytoplasmic components, under normal circumstances is as follows:

- naturally occurring specific IgM aabs will assist in the removal of intracytoplasmic ags prior to being digested into reusable small MW peptides in mononuclear cells [7, 20, 21, 69, 103, 104]. This physiological process prevents toxic accumulation and/or possible chemical/structural modification of self ags that could lead to pathogenic IgG aab production resulting in an autoimmune disease.;
- some of the released aags *per se* will stimulate production of specific IgM aabs and some of the released aags will combine with specific IgM aabs to form ICs. ICs (released intracytoplasmic self ag X homologous anti-released intracytoplasmic self ag IgM aab) further stimulate, more specifically produced IgM aabs and maintain constant levels of specific IgM aabs in the circulation (secondary immune response).;

The specific intracytoplasmic ag clearing IgM aabs fulfill a physiological role and by efficiently removing cellular breakdown products from the system they significantly contribute to tolerance to self [15, 17]. However, if massive release of an intracytoplasmic ag occurs, because of injury to a target ag of cells located eg. in an organ, then the available and produced IgM aabs might not be sufficient enough to efficiently and in a timely manner clear the cellular breakdown products from the system. In this case, the lingering ags (if modifying agents are present in the system) could become structurally or chemically modified. Such modified ags could produce pathogenic IgG aabs and initiate and maintain an autoimmune disease.

There are several opinions how pathogenic IgG aab response is initiated and maintained. In our opinion, autoimmune diseases as observed in experimental autoimmune disease models (and most likely in naturally occurring autoimmune diseases of humans as well) eg. HN and SPHN are initiated and maintained by repeated exposure/injections of modified self ags (eg. rKF3 ag in FCA; azo-rKF3 ag in FCA [51]; rKF3 in Alum [14]; azo-rKF3 [16] etc.). When a modified self ag, like a hapten-self protein conjugate (eg. azo-rKF3 ag), is presented to immune cells it is processed not quite as a self ag and a pathogenic IgG aab is produced against it. Such an aab is a cross-reactive aab. It is able to react with the ag that initiated its production (i.e., the azo-rKF3 ag) but also with the native ag (i.e., the rKF3 ag) which is an integral part of the BB zone of cells of the renal convoluted tubules and also located (but not produced) in the glomeruli. This cross-reactive IgG aab will cause the autoimmune disease by damaging the BB zone of cells of the renal proximal convoluted tubules. The released nephritogenic ag from the BB will get into the circulation and contributes to further stimulation/production of IgM aabs and to layered deposition of ICs in the glomeruli, together with the pathogenic anti-HN ag IgG aab and complement components, causing MGN [Figure 3].

During the course of the autoimmune disease SPHN both pathogenic IgG and non-pathogenic IgM aabs are present in the circulation [14, 15, 17]. The pathogenic IgG aabs cause irreversible damage to the target organ by continuously bombarding/damaging the nephritogenic ag in the BB of the renal proximal convoluted tubules and also by contributing to IC deposition in the glomeruli (exacerbation). The IgM aabs, also being cross-reactive aabs, aim to minimize/terminate autoimmune disease causing events (remission). However, as long as the pathogenic IgG aab producing cell lines are stimulated by the modified nephritogenic ag *per se* or in the form of ICs [modified nephritogenic ag X rat anti-rat modified nephritogenic ag IgG aab], and during the chronic progressive phase of the autoimmune disease by the native nephritogenic ag containing ICs as well [native nephritogenic ag X rat anti-rat modified nephritogenic ag IgG aab], the autoimmune disease causing events will progress [14, 15, 17]. The pathogenic IgG aab producing nephritogenic ags must be removed from the circulation to halt (terminate) autoimmune disease causing immune events. Presently employed medical interventions, using immunosuppressive agents, monoclonal abs etc. cannot achieve termination of such events. They can somewhat interfere with the production of pathogenic IgG aabs by targeting the ab producing cell lines non-specifically, and in the meantime cause undesirable side effects.

Barabas and colleagues introduced a new vaccination method – the third way of immunizing after active and passive immunizations – that allows an endogenous ag initiated and maintained autoimmune disease, by pathogenic aabs, prophylactically (to prevent) and therapeutically remedy (terminate) specifically and without side effects [8, 9, 12, 13, 18]. To our knowledge this was the first time that an endogenous ag caused pathogenic immune response was down regulated without the use of drugs by the immune system's natural abilities to correct harmful immune responses (after providing the necessary information) that targeted normal structural and functional parts of the affected animal's kidney. In order to prevent or terminate SPHN in rats, the modified nephritogenic ag has to be neutralized/removed from the system. It can be achieved by specifically increasing IgM aabs in the circulation against the native nephritogenic ag [15, 17]. We have produced nephritogenic ag (rKF3 ag) and homologous IgM ab against the nephritogenic ag (rarKF3 ag IgM ab) and thereafter produced ICs at slight ag access for injections [rKF3 ag X rarKF3 ag IgM ab] rKF3. The injected IC in SPHN rats increased the production of the same ab with the same specificity against the target ag that was present in the IC, namely rarKF3 ag IgM aab. Since the developing IgM aab was cross-reactive it was able to assist in the removal of both native and modified rKF3 ags from the circulation. In the absence of the pathogenic IgG aab producing ag in the circulation the pathogenic IgG aab cell lines were no longer stimulated and pathogenic immune responses targeting the BB cells of the renal proximal convoluted tubules and the glomeruli localized nephritogenic ag were halted. Measurements of both pathogenic IgG aab and non-pathogenic IgM aab responses against the BB localized nephritogenic ag by the indirect fluorescence ab test clearly revealed the cessation of pathogenic immune responses [15, 17]. At this stage the G/M ratio was zero [17], indicating the absence of IgG aabs in the circulation against the target nephritogenic ag.

We believe implicated pathogenic immune responses, which initiate and maintain most autoimmune diseases, can be prevented and also terminated with appropriate application of the MVT specifically and without side effects, achieving regained tolerance to self.

Table 1. Immune responses against exogenous and endogenous ags

	Exposure of the cells of the immune system to exogenous/endogenous ags	Immune initiated response	Results in:	Immune response that could neutralize/eliminate exogenous and endogenous disease causing ags from the host's internal environment is the best approach by the intervention of:
Exogenous ags	Continuous bombardment of the immune system by bacteria, viruses, toxins etc. Infectious/contagious disease causing agents result in disease. Occasional mutant bacteria/virus can cause serious outbreaks of contagious diseases (eg. influenza).	Cell and humoral ab response. Cell and humoral ab response. Often delayed.	Neutralization or clearance of infectious/toxic agents. Neutralization or clearance of infectious/toxic agents. Serious illness/death.	Innate and adaptive immunity. Prophylactic vaccination. Passive immunization.MVT.

Table 1. (Continued)

Endogenous ags	Under 'normal' conditions endogenous ags do not cause disease. Self ags modified chemically/structurally; molecules similar to self (molecular mimicry). Cells with cancer specific ags on their outer cell membranes.	Cellular breakdown products are assisted in their removal by specific IgM aabs prior to being degraded in mononuclear cells. IgM aabs are health promoting abs. Can cause cell mediated and/or humoral aab responses. Cancer specific ags are small MW ags being integral parts of cell membranes (not recognized often as non-self). Immune response against cancer cells is often incomplete.	Maintenance of tolerance to self. Autoimmune diseases. Cancer.	Naturally occurring IgM aabs and mononuclear cells. MVT. Passive immunization (presently).

The cells of the immune system face two groups of ags: 1. those that come from the external environment; and 2. those that come from the internal environment. A well functioning immune system maintains tolerance to self by removing/neutralizing ags that are non-self (i.e., bacteria, viruses, toxins, modified self ags etc.). However, when the immune system is overwhelmed eg. by a modified endogenous ag, an autoimmune disease can occur; and when the system is compromised cancer can emerge.

Abbreviations: aab, autoantibody; ab, antibody; ag, antigen; MVT, modified vaccination technique; MW, molecular weight.

ACKNOWLEDGMENTS

We acknowledge the assistance of our research associate, Zoltan B. Kovacs, in computer and laboratory-related work.

REFERENCES

[1] Agmon-Levin N., Paz Z., Israeli E., Shoenfeld Y. Vaccines and autoimmunity. *Nat. Rev. Rheumatol.*, 2009, 5, 648-52.

[2] Alballa S., Fritzler M., Davis P. A. case of drug induced lupus due to carbamazepine. *J. Rheumatol.*, 1987, 14, 599-600.

[3] Alousi MA., Post RS., Heymann W. Experimental autoimmune nephrosis in rats. Morphogenesis of the glomerular lesion: immunohistochemical and electron microscopic studies. *Am. J. Pathol.*, 1969, 54, 47-71.

[4] Andreakos E., Taylor PC., Feldmann M. Monoclonal antibodies in immune and inflammatory diseases. *Curr. Opin. Biotechnol.,* 2002, 13, 615-20.

[5] Andres G., Brentjens JR., Caldwell PR., Camussi G., Matsuo S. Formation of immune deposits and disease. *Lab Invest*, 1986, 55, 510-20.

[6] Arbuckle MR., McClain MT., Rubertone MV., Scofield RH; Dennis GJ., James JA. et al. Development of autoantibodies before the clinical onset of systemic lupus erythematosus. *N. Engl. J. Med.,* 2003, 349, 1526-33.

[7] Avrameas S. Natural autoantibodies: from 'horror autotoxicus' to 'gnothi seauton'. *Immunol Today,* 1991, 12, 154-9.

[8] Barabas AZ., Cole CD., Barabas AD., Bahlis NJ., Lafreniere R. New vaccination technology for endogenous antigen-derived ailments. *IDrugs,* 2008, 11, 111-5.

[9] Barabas AZ., Cole CD., Barabas AD., Bahlis NJ., Lafreniere R. A. vaccination technique to combat presently untreatable chronic ailments. *BioProcessing Journal*, 2007, 6, 12-8.

[10] Barabas AZ., Cole CD., Barabas AD., Barabas AN., Lafreniere R. Reduced incidence of slowly progressive Heymann nephritis in rats immunized with a modified vaccination technique. *Clin. Dev. Immunol.,* 2006, 13, 17-24.

[11] Barabas AZ., Cole CD., Barabas AD., Cowan JM., Yoon CS., Waisman DM et al. Presence of immunoglobulin M antibodies *around the*

*glomer*ular capillaries and in the mesangium of normal and passive Heymann nephritis rats. *Int. J. Exp. Pathol.,* 2004, 85, 201-12.

[12] Barabas AZ., Cole CD., Barabas AD., Graeff RM., Lafreniere R., Weir DM. Correcting autoimmune anomalies in autoimmune disorders by immunological means, employing the modified vaccination technique. *Autoimmun. Rev.,* 2009, 8, 552-7.

[13] Barabas AZ., Cole CD., Barabas AD., Graeff RM., Lafreniere R., Weir DM. Modified vaccination technique for prophylactic and therapeutic applications to combat endogenous antigen-induced disorders. *Scandinavian Journal of Immunology,* 2010, 71, 125-33.

[14] Barabas AZ., Cole CD., Barabas AD., Lafreniere R. Production of a new model of slowly progressive Heymann nephritis. *Int. J. Exp. Pathol.,* 2003, 84, 245-58.

[15] Barabas AZ., Cole CD., Barabas AD., Lafreniere R. Down-regulation of pathogenic autoantibody response in a slowly progressive Heymann nephritis kidney disease model. *Int. J. Exp. Pathol.,* 2004, 85, 321-34.

[16] Barabas AZ., Cole CD., Barabas AD., Lafreniere R. Production of Heymann nephritis by a chemically modified renal antigen. *Int. J. Exp. Pathol.,* 2004, 85, 277-85.

[17] Barabas AZ., Cole CD., Barabas AD., Lafreniere R. Downregulation of a pathogenic autoantibody response by IgM autoantibodies directed against the nephritogenic antigen in slowly progressive Heymann nephritis. *Pathol. Int.,* 2006, 56, 181-90.

[18] Barabas AZ., Cole CD., Barabas AD., Lafreniere R. A. modified vaccination technique for the prevention and treatment of an experimental autoimmune kidney disease. *Ann. N. Y. Acad. Sci.,* 2007, 1110, 619-29.

[19] Barabas AZ., Cole CD., Barabas AD., Lafreniere R. Preventative and therapeutic vaccination to combat an experimental autoimmune kidney disease. *Biologics: Targets and Therapy,* 2007, 1, 59-68.

[20] Barabas AZ., Cole CD., Barabas AD., Lafreniere R. An experimental autoimmune kidney disease caused by pathogenic autoantibodies. In Petrelli C, editor. *New research on autoantibodies*. Hauppauge NY: Nova Science Publishers, Inc., 2008, 151-72.

[21] Barabas AZ., Cole CD., Barabas AD., Lafreniere R. Pathogenic and nonpathogenic autoimmune events – the good and/or the bad? In Dubois Q, editor. *Autoantibodies research progress*. Hauppauge NY: Nova Science Publishers, Inc., 2008, 9-18.

[22] Barabas AZ., Cole CD, Kovacs ZB., Lafreniere R. Elevated antibody response by antigen presentation in immune complexes. *Med. Sci. Monit.,* 2007, 13, BR119-BR124.

[23] Barabas AZ., Cole CD., Lafreniere R., Weir DM. A new vaccination method for exogenous and endogenous antigen initiated disorders. In Bezio AI, Campbell BE, editors. *Vaccinations: Procedures, Types and Controversy*. Hauppauge NY: Nova Science Publishers, Inc., 2012, 1-25.

[24] Barabas AZ., Cole CD., Weir DM., Lafreniere R. Immunopathological events in an experimental autoimmune kidney disease and how those events can be terminated to regain tolerance to self. In Petrov M, editor. *Autoimmune disorders: symptoms, diagnosis and treatment*. Hauppauge NY: Nova Science Publishers, Inc., 2011, 35-66.

[25] Barabas AZ., Cole CD., Weir DM., Lafreniere R. The primary target antigenic site in Heymann nephritis is the renal proximal convoluted tubules' brush border associated zone of cells. In Petrov M, editor. *Autoimmune Disorders: Symptoms, Diagnosis and Treatment.* Hauppauge NY: Nova Science Publishers, Inc., 2011, 281-92.

[26] Barabas AZ., Lafreniere R. Antigen-specific down-regulation of immunopathological events in an experimental autoimmune kidney disease. *Autoimmun. Rev.,* 2005, 4, 565-70.

[27] Barabas AZ., Lannigan R. Auto-immune nephritis in rats. *J. Pathol.,* 1969, 97, 537-43.

[28] Barabas AZ., Nagi AH., Lannigan R., Womersley RA. The effect of cortisone treatment on autologous immune complex glomerulonephritis in rats. *Br. J. Exp. Pathol.,* 1970, 51, 541-6.

[29] Batsford SR., Weghaupt R., Takamiya H., Vogt A. Studies on the mesangial handling of protein antigens: influence of size, charge and biologic activity. *Nephron,* 1985, 41, 146-51.

[30] Bhan AK., Schneeberger EE., Baird LG., Collins AB., Kamata K., Bradford D et al. Studies with monoclonal antibodies against brush border antigens in Heymann nephritis. *Lab Invest,* 1985, 53, 421-32.

[31] Blank M., Shoenfeld Y. B cell targeted therapy in autoimmunity. *J. Autoimmun.,* 2007, 28, 62-8.

[32] Boes M., Schmidt T., Linkemann K., Beaudette BC., Marshak-Rothstein A., Chen J. Accelerated development of IgG autoantibodies and autoimmune disease in the absence of secreted IgM. *Proc. Natl. Acad. Sci. US,* 2000, 97, 1184-9.

[33] Byrd JC., Waselenko JK., Maneatis TJ., Murphy T., Ward FT., Monahan BP et al. Rituximab therapy in hematologic malignancy patients with

circulating blood tumor cells: association with increased infusion-related side effects and rapid blood tumor clearance. *J. Clin. Oncol.,* 1999, 17, 791-5.

[34] Challice J., Barabas AZ., Cornish J., Bruce JW., Lannigan R. Passive Heymann nephritis in pre- and post-natal rats. *Br. J. Exp. Pathol.,* 1986, 67, 915-24.

[35] Chastain EM., Miller SD. Molecular mimicry as an inducing trigger for CNS autoimmune demyelinating disease. *Immunol. Rev.,* 2012, 245, 227-38.

[36] Disis ML., Shiota FM., Cheever MA. Human HER-2/neu protein immunization circumvents tolerance to rat neu: a vaccine strategy for 'self' tumour antigens. *Immunology,* 1998, 93, 192-9.

[37] Dorner T., Radbruch A., Burmester GR. B-cell-directed therapies for autoimmune disease. *Nat. Rev. Rheumatol.,* 2009, 5, 433-41.

[38] Ebringer A. Molecular mimicry as the basis of a new theory of autoimmunity. In Zouali M, editor. *Frontiers in Autoimmunity: fundamental aspects and clinical perspectives*. Amsterdam Netherlands: IOS Press, 2003, 79-99.

[39] Ebringer A., Thorpe C., Pirt J., Wilson C., Cunningham P., Ettelaie C. Bovine spongiform encephalopathy: is it an autoimmune disease due to bacteria showing molecular mimicry with brain antigens? *Environ. Health Perspect.,* 1997, 105, 1172-4.

[40] Edgington TS., Glassock RJ., Dixon FJ. Autologous immune complex nephritis induced with renal tubular antigen. I. Identification and isolation of the pathogenetic antigen. *J. Exp. Med.,* 1968, 127, 555-72.

[41] Edgington TS., Glassock RJ., Watson JI., Dixon FJ. Characterization and isolation of specific renal tubular epithelial antigens. *J. Immunol.,* 1967, 99, 1199-210.

[42] Feldmann M., Steinman L. Design of effective immunotherapy for human autoimmunity. *Nature,* 2005, 435, 612-9.

[43] Ghaussy NO., Sibbitt WL., Jr.; Qualls CR. Cigarette smoking, alcohol consumption, and the risk of systemic lupus erythematosus: a case-control study. *J. Rheumatol.*, 2001, 28, 2449-53.

[44] Glassock RJ. The pathogenesis of idiopathic membranous nephropathy: a 50-year odyssey. *Am. J. Kidney Dis.,* 2010, 56, 157-67.

[45] Glassock RJ., Edgington TS., Watson JI., Dixon FJ. Autologous immune complex nephritis induced with renal tubular antigen. II. The pathogenetic mechanism. *J. Exp. Med.,* 1968, 127, 573-88.

[46] Gonzalez-Cabrero J., de Nicolas R., Ortiz A., Mampaso F., Hernando L., Egido J. Presence of circulating antibodies against brush border antigens (Fx1A) in a patient with membranous nephropathy and bilateral pyeloureteral stenosis. Comparison with idiopathic membranous nephropathy. *Nephrol. Dial. Transplant.,* 1992, 7, 293-9.

[47] Greenwald P., Clifford CK., Milner JA. Diet and cancer prevention. *Eur. J. Cancer,* 2001, 37, 948-65.

[48] Grupe WE; Kaplan MH. Demonstration of an antibody to proximal tubular antigen in the pathogenesis of experimental autoimmune nephrosis in rats. *J Lab Clin Med,* 1969, 74, 400-9.

[49] Gullstrand B., Martensson U., Sturfelt G., Bengtsson AA., Truedsson L. Complement classical pathway components are all important in clearance of apoptotic and secondary necrotic cells. *Clin. Exp. Immunol.,* 2009, 156, 303-11.

[50] Heymann W., Hackel DB., Harwood S., Wilson SG., Hunter JLP. Production of nephritic syndrome in rats by Freund's adjuvant and rat kidney suspensions. *Proc. Soc. Exp. Biol. Med.,* 1959, 100, 660-4.

[51] Heymann W., Kmetec EP., Wilson SG., Hunter JLP., Hackel DB., Cuppage F. Experimental autoimmune renal disease in rats. In Grabar P, Miescher PA, editors. *IIIrd International Symposium of Immunopathology*. Switzerland: Schwabe and Co., Basel, 1963, 240-51.

[52] Hogan SL., Muller KE., Jennette JC., Falk RJ. A review of therapeutic studies of idiopathic membranous glomerulopathy. *Am. J. Kidney Dis.,* 1995, 25, 862-75.

[53] Jiang X., Khursigara G., Rubin RL. Transformation of lupus-inducing drugs to cytotoxic products by activated neutrophils. *Science,* 1994, 266, 810-3.

[54] Kamata K., Baird LG., Erikson ME., Collins AB., McCluskey RT. Characterization of antigens and antibody specificities involved in Heymann nephritis. *J. Immunol.,* 1985, 135, 2400-8.

[55] Kerjaschki D. Molecular development of immune deposits and proteinuria in Heymann nephritis. *Clin. Investig.,* 1993, 71, 817-21.

[56] Kerjaschki D. Pathogenetic concepts of membranous glomerulopathy (MGN). *J. Nephrol. 2000,* 2000, 13, S96-100.

[57] Kerjaschki D., Farquhar MG. The pathogenic antigen of Heymann nephritis is a membrane glycoprotein of the renal proximal tubule brush border. *Proc. Natl. Acad. Sci. US,* 1982, 79, 5557-81.

[58] Kerjaschki D., Farquhar MG. Immunocytochemical localization of the Heymann nephritis antigen (GP330) in glomerular epithelial cells of normal Lewis rats. *J. Exp. Med.,* 1983, 157, 667-86.

[59] Kerjaschki D., Neale TJ. Molecular mechanisms of glomerular injury in rat experimental membranous nephropathy (Heymann nephritis). *J. Am. Soc. Nephrol.*, 1996, 7, 2518-26.

[60] Lannigan R., Barabas AZ., Peters K., Hardwick J. Some experimental models of the nephrotic syndrome. In Bajusz E, Jasmin G, editors. *Meth. Achievment Experimental Pathology*. New York: Karger, Basel, 1969, 141-70.

[61] Leandro MJ., Edwards JC., Cambridge G; Ehrenstein MR., Isenberg DA. An open study of B lymphocyte depletion in systemic lupus erythematosus. *Arthritis. Rheum.*, 2002, 46, 2673-7.

[62] Lin TS. Novel agents in chronic lymphocytic leukemia: efficacy and tolerability of new therapies. *Clin. Lymphoma Myeloma,* 2008, 8 Suppl 4, S137-S143.

[63] Lollini PL., Forni G. Antitumor vaccines: is it possible to prevent a tumor? *Cancer Immunol. Immunother.*, 2002, 51, 409-16.

[64] Manson JJ., Mauri C., Ehrenstein MR. Natural serum IgM maintains immunological homeostasis and prevents autoimmunity. *Springer Semin. Immunopathol.,* 2005, 26, 425-32.

[65] Manz RA., Arce S., Cassese G., Hauser AE,. Hiepe F., Radbruch A. Humoral immunity and long-lived plasma cells. *Curr. Opin. Immunol.,* 2002, 14, 517-21.

[66] Marr LA., Gilham DE., Campbell JD., Fraser AR. Immunology in the clinic review series; focus on cancer: double trouble for tumours: bi-functional and redirected T cells as effective cancer immunotherapies. *Clin. Exp. Immunol.,* 2012, 167, 216-25.

[67] Matsukawa W., Hara S., Yoshida F., Suzuki N., Fukatsu A., Yuzawa Y et al. Effects of a new immunosuppressive agent, FK506, in rats with active Heymann nephritis. *J. Lab Clin. Med.,* 1992, 119, 116-23.

[68] Mendrick DL., Noble B., Brentjens JR., Andres GA. Antibody-mediated injury to proximal tubules in Heymann nephritis. *Kidney Int.,* 1980, 18, 328-43.

[69] Mevorach D., Mascarenhas JO., Gershov D., Elkon KB. Complement-dependent clearance of apoptotic cells by human macrophages. *J. Exp. Med.,* 1998, 188, 2313-20.

[70] Mokhtarian F., Zhang Z., Shi Y., Gonzales E., Sobel RA. Molecular mimicry between a viral peptide and a myelin oligodendrocyte

glycoprotein peptide induces autoimmune demyelinating disease in mice. *J. Neuroimmunol.,* 1999, 95, 43-54.

[71] Molina V., Shoenfeld Y. Infection, vaccines and other environmental triggers of autoimmunity. *Autoimmunity,* 2005, 38, 235-45.

[72] Naruse T., Fukasawa T., Hirokawa N., Oike S., Miyakawa Y. The pathogenesis of experimental membranous glomerulonephritis induced with homologous nephritogenic tubular antigen. *J. Exp. Med.,* 1976, 144, 1347-62.

[73] Naruse T., Fukasawa T., Miyakawa Y. Laboratory model of membranous glomerulonephritis in rats induced by pronase-digested homologous renal tubular epithelial antigen. *Lab Invest,* 1975, 33, 141-6.

[74] Neale TJ., Couser WG., Salant DJ., Lowenstein LM., Wilson CB. Specific uptake of Heymann's nephritic kidney eluate by rat kidney: studies in vivo and in isolated perfused kidneys. *Lab Invest,* 1982, 46, 450-3.

[75] Noble B., Van Liew JB., Brentjens JR., Andres GA. Effect of reimmunization with Fx1A late in the course of Heymann nephritis. *Lab Invest,* 1982, 47, 427-36.

[76] Ogden CA; Kowalewski R; Peng Y; Montenegro V; Elkon KB. IgM is required for efficient complement mediated phagocytosis of apoptotic cells in vivo. *Autoimmunity,* 2005, 38, 259-64.

[77] Orbach H., Shoenfeld Y. Vaccination infection and autoimmunity: myth and reality VIAMR 2005-10-26-28, Beau-Rivage Palace Hotel, LaUSnne, Switzerland. *Autoimmun. Rev.,* 2007, 6, 261-6.

[78] Orlando RA., Farquhar MG. Identification of a cell line that expresses a cell surface and a soluble form of the gp330/receptor-associated protein (RAP) Heymann nephritis antigenic complex. *Proc. Natl. Acad. Sci. US,* 1993, 90, 4082-6.

[79] Perna A., Schieppati A., Zamora J., Giuliano GA., Braun N., Remuzzi G. Immunosuppressive treatment for idiopathic membranous nephropathy: a systematic review. *Am. J. Kidney Dis.,* 2004, 44, 385-401.

[80] Perosa F., Favoino E., Caragnano MA., Prete M., Dammacco F. CD20: a target antigen for immunotherapy of autoimmune diseases. *Autoimmun. Rev.*, 2005, 4, 526-31.

[81] Pinckard RN., Weir DM. Antibodies against the mitochondrial fraction of liver after toxic liver damage in rats. *Clin. Exp. Immunol.*, 1966, 1, 33-43.

[82] Quartier P., Potter PK., Ehrenstein MR., Walport MJ., Botto M. Predominant role of IgM-dependent activation of the classical pathway in the clearance of dying cells by murine bone marrow-derived macrophages in vitro. *Eur. J. Immunol.,* 2005, 35, 252-60.

[83] Radbruch A., Muehlinghaus G., Luger EO., Inamine A., Smith KG., Dorner T et al. Competence and competition: the challenge of becoming a long-lived plasma cell. *Nat. Rev. Immunol.,* 2006, 6, 741-50.

[84] Raychowdhury R., Zheng G., Brown D., McCluskey RT. Induction of Heymann nephritis with a gp330/megalin fusion protein. *Am. J. Pathol.,* 1996, 148, 1613-23.

[85] Robinson MK., Shaller C., Garmestani K., Plascjak PS., Hodge KM., Yuan QA et al. Effective treatment of established human breast tumor xenografts in immunodeficient mice with a single dose of the alpha-emitting radioisotope astatine-211 conjugated to anti-HER2/neu diabodies. *Clin. Cancer Res.,* 2008, 14, 875-82.

[86] Ronco P., Debiec H. Target antigens and nephritogenic antibodies in membranous nephropathy: of rats and men. *Semin. Immunopathol.,* 2007, 29, 445-58.

[87] Ronco P., Debiec H. Antigen identification in membranous nephropathy moves toward targeted monitoring and new therapy. *J. Am. Soc. Nephrol.,* 2010, 21, 564-9.

[88] Ronco P., Neale TJ., Wilson CB., Galceran M., Verroust P. An immunopathologic study of a 330-kD protein defined by monoclonal antibodies and reactive with anti-RTE alpha 5 antibodies and kidney eluates from active Heymann nephritis. *J. Immunol.,* 1986, 136, 125-30.

[89] Schulze C., Munoz LE., Franz S., Sarter K., Chaurio RA., Gaipl US et al. Clearance deficiency--a potential link between infections and autoimmunity. *Autoimmun. Rev.,* 2008, 8, 5-8.

[90] Shoenfeld Y., Gilburd B., Abu-Shakra M., Amital H., Barzilai O., Berkun Y et al. The mosaic of autoimmunity: genetic factors involved in autoimmune diseases--2008. *Isr. Med. Assoc. J.,* 2008, 10, 3-7.

[91] Shoenfeld Y., Zandman-Goddard G., Stojanovich L., Cutolo M., Amital H., Levy Y et al. The mosaic of autoimmunity: hormonal and environmental factors involved in autoimmune diseases--2008. *Isr. Med. Assoc. J.,* 2008, 10, 8-12.

[92] Singh AK., Makker SP. Circulatory antigens of Heymann nephritis. I. Identification and partial characterization. *Immunology,* 1986, 57, 467-72.

[93] Singh AK., Schwartz MM. Circulatory antigen of Heymann nephritis. II. Isolation of a 70,000 MW antigen from normal rat serum which cross-reacts with Heymann nephritis antigen. *Immunology,* 1986, 59, 451-8.
[94] Totoritis MC., Rubin RL. Drug-induced lupus. Genetic, clinical, and laboratory features. *Postgrad. Med.,* 1985, 78, 149-61.
[95] Tsukada Y., Ono K., Maezawa A., Yano S., Naruse T. A major pathogenic antigen of Heymann nephritis is present exclusively in the renal proximal tubule brush border--studies with a monoclonal antibody against pronase-digested tubular antigen. *Clin. Exp. Immunol.,* 1994, 96, 303-10.
[96] Waldner H. The role of innate immune responses in autoimmune disease development. *Autoimmun. Rev.*, 2009, 8, 400-4.
[97] Weir DM. Immunological reaction after tissue injury. *Lancet,* 1964, 1, 749-50.
[98] Weir DM. The immune response after tissue injury. *Pathol. Eur.,* 1966, 1, 108-18.
[99] Weir DM. The immunologicial consequences of cell death. *Lancet,* 1967, 2, 1071-3.
[100] Weir DM. Altered antigens and autoimmunity. *Vox. Sang.,* 1969, 16, 304-13.
[101] Weir DM; Elson CJ. Antitissue antibodies and immunological tolerance to self. *Arthritis Rheum.,* 1969, 12, 254-60.
[102] Weir DM., Pinckard RN. Failure to induce tolerance to rat tissue antigens. *Immunology,* 1967, 13, 373-80.
[103] Weir DM., Pinckard RN., Elson CJ.,Suckling DE. Naturally occurring anti-tissue antibodies in rat sera. *Clin. Exp. Immunol.*, 1966, 1, 433-42.
[104] Wermeling F., Karlsson MC., McGaha TL. An anatomical view on macrophages in tolerance. *Autoimmun. Rev.*, 2009, 9, 49-52.
[105] Wucherpfennig KW. Mechanisms for the induction of autoimmunity by infectious agents. *J. Clin. Invest.,* 2001, 108, 1097-104.
[106] Yoshida T., Mei H; Dorner T., Hiepe F., Radbruch A., Fillatreau S et al. Memory B and memory plasma cells. *Immunol. Rev.,* 2010, 237, 117-39.
[107] Yung RL., Johnson KJ., Richardson BC. New concepts in the pathogenesis of drug-induced lupus. *Lab Invest,* 1995, 73, 746-59.

In: Autoantibodies
Editors: G. E. Jenkins and J. I. Hall
ISBN: 978-1-62081-560-1

Chapter II

ANTI-FACTOR H AUTOANTIBODIES IN KIDNEY DISEASE: DETECTION, PATHOGENIC ROLE AND RELEVANCE FOR TREATMENT

Mihály Józsi
Junior Research Group Cellular Immunobiology,
Leibniz Institute for Natural Product Research and Infection Biology – Hans Knöll Institute, Jena, Germany

ABSTRACT

Complement is an essential humoral component of the innate immune system. It participates in various physiological processes including the destruction of pathogens, waste disposal, inflammation, modulation of the activation of innate and adaptive immune cells, and tissue regeneration. The complement system consists of more than forty soluble and membrane-bound proteins, which form three major activation pathways and a terminal complement pathway, regulate the system and mediate biological functions such as cell activation. Complement deficiencies and malfunctions are associated with various infectious, inflammatory and immune disorders. Dysregulation of the alternative complement pathway is involved in the pathogenesis of the kidney diseases atypical hemolytic uremic syndrome and dense deposit disease. Factor H is a major inhibitor of the alternative complement pathway. Certain factor H mutations and autoantibodies against this regulatory protein are associated with atypical hemolytic uremic syndrome and dense deposit disease. The anti-factor H autoantibody-associated forms of these diseases require a corresponding treatment. This review provides an overview of the main factor H functions and the role of anti-factor H autoantibodies in kidney diseases. Furthermore, the problems of anti-factor H autoantibody detection, studies on the functional relevance and potential pathogenicity of such autoantibodies, and the importance of prompt autoantibody detection for the selection of appropriate treatment for the affected patients are discussed.

INTRODUCTION

The complement system is an important humoral arm of innate immunity, with functions in host defense against infections, host-nonhost discrimination, clearance of immune complexes and apoptotic/necrotic cells, tissue remodelling, and regulation of the adaptive immune response (Ricklin et al., 2010). Complement is composed of more than forty molecules, which recognize targets, propagate the complement cascade, regulate this system or mediate cellular functions. Complement is activated through three major pathways, the classical, lectin and alternative pathways (**Figure 1**). The classical pathway is activated by immunoglobulins and pentraxins, the lectin pathway is activated by repetitive microbial carbohydrate groups and acetylated groups, and the alternative pathway is constantly activated at a low rate by the hydrolysis of the thioester bond of the C3 molecule. After the initial recognition and activation steps, a C3 convertase enzyme is assembled that cleaves C3 into C3a and C3b. C3b is an opsonin and it further propagates the cascade by forming additional C3 convertases and, via binding to C3 convertases, by forming the C5 convertases. The latter initiate the terminal pathway by cleaving C5. The terminal complement pathway may eventually lead to the formation of the C5b-9 membrane attack complex, which punches holes in target cell membranes and thus causes osmotic lysis.

While the activation of this innate effector system is required to destroy pathogens, efficient regulation is important to prevent damage of by-stander host cells and tissues. This protection is ensured by a number of complement regulators, both in fluid-phase and on cell- and tissue surfaces. Improper complement regulation may result in excessive complement activation on self-tissue and lead to disease, such as the kidney diseases atypical hemolytic uremic syndrome and dense deposit disease. Because the alternative pathway is always activated and it amplifies complement activation secondary to the initiation of the classical and lectin pathways, its proper regulation is particularly important (Zipfel et al., 2006).

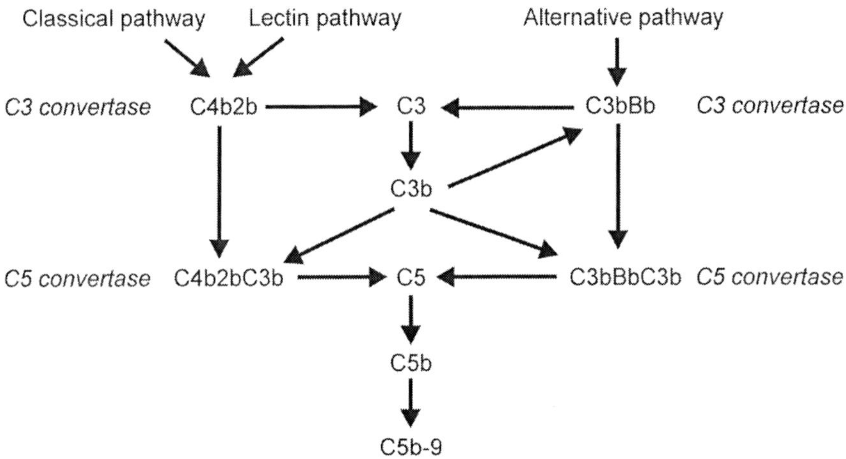

Figure 1. Schematic overview of the main complement pathways.

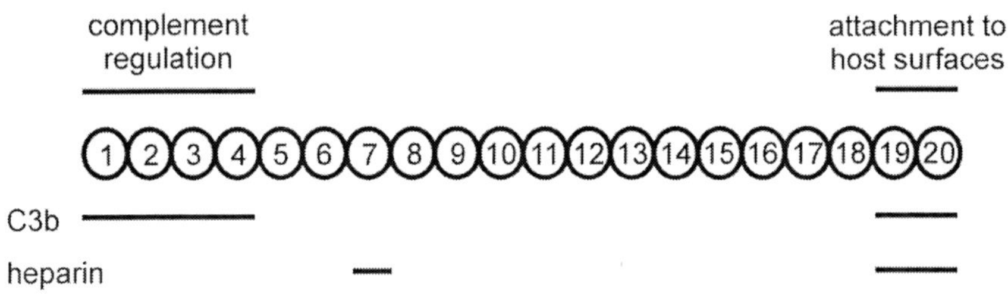

Figure 2. Schematic structure of factor H. Factor H is composed of 20 SCRs. SCRs 1-4 mediate the complement regulatory functions of factor H, whereas SCRs 19-20 mediate factor H attachment to host cell surfaces. The main C3b and heparin/glycosaminoglycan binding sites are indicated by horizontal lines under the respective domains.

FACTOR H

Factor H is the major regulator of the alternative complement pathway (Kopp et al., 2012). Factor H is a 150-kDa glycoprotein with a plasma concentration of approximately 250 μg/ml. It is composed of 20 short consensus repeat (SCR) domains (also termed complement control protein modules, CCP) (**Figure 2**).

Factor H serves as a cofactor for the inactivation of C3b by factor I, prevents the formation of the alternative pathway C3bBb convertase by competing with factor B for C3b binding, and facilitates the decay of the C3bBb convertase (Weiler et al., 1976; Whaley and Ruddy, 1976; Pangburn et al., 1977). These complement regulatory functions are mediated by SCRs 1-4 at the N-terminus of the molecule (Gordon et al., 1995; Kühn et al., 1995; Kühn and Zipfel, 1996; Wu et al., 2009). In addition to its complement inhibitory action in the fluid phase (i.e., in body fluids), factor H can also attach to basement membranes and host cells and inhibit complement activation on these surfaces (Józsi et al., 2004). For this function the C-terminal SCRs 19-20 are critical (Meri and Pangburn, 1990; Pangburn 2000, 2002; Ferreira et al., 2006; Józsi et al., 2007a). These domains contain binding sites for C3b and C3d and also for heparin / cell surface glycosaminoglycans (Sharma and Pangburn, 1996; Blackmore et al., 1998; Jokiranta et al. 2000, 2005). The presence of polyanionic molecules, such as glycosaminoglycans and sialic acid, on host cells allows factor H to discriminate between host and nonhost surfaces. Recent structural studies revealed the exact binding sites for C3b/C3d and polyanionic molecules within SCRs 19-20 (Kajander et al., 2011; Morgan et al., 2011). In addition to normal host cells, factor H binds and prevents excessive complement activation on apoptotic cells and presumably on basement membranes and extracellular matrix (Trouw et al., 2007; Clark et al., 2010; Didangelos et al., 2010).

Functional impairment of factor H or inefficient interaction of factor H with host structures may result in a compromized control of alternative pathway activation. Factor H dysfunction is associated with several diseases including age-related macular degeneration (AMD), atypical hemolytic uremic syndrome (aHUS) and dense deposit disease (DDD). Mutations and polymorphisms in the factor H gene (*CFH*), as well as genomic rearrangements affecting the *CFH* gene and in its direct vicinity the related *CFHR* genes have been described in these diseases (Józsi and Zipfel, 2008). In addition to the genetic defects, autoantibodies to factor H as an acquired (autoimmune) abnormality are detected in some aHUS and DDD patients.

ANTI-FACTOR H AUTOANTIBODIES

Autoantibodies to complement components are described in several diseases, such as anti-C1q antibodies in systemic lupus erythematosus, anti-C1 inhibitor autoantibodies in patients with acquired angioedema and C3 nephritic factor in membranoproliferative glomerulonephritis type I, type III, dense deposit disease and partial lipodystrophy (Trouw et al., 2001). Thus far, anti-factor H autoantibodies have been detected in a few diseases only, as discussed below.

Anti-Factor H Autoantibodies in Atypical Hemolytic Uremic Syndrome

Anti-factor H autoantibodies are detected in approximately 10% of the patients diagnosed with aHUS (Skerka et al., 2009). aHUS is a severe and rare kidney disease characterized by Coombs-negative hemolytic anemia, thrombocytopenia and acute renal impairment (Noris and Remuzzi, 2009). aHUS is also a disease characterized by impaired alternative complement pathway regulation. Mutations and polymorphisms are described in several complement genes in aHUS-patients (Loirat and Frémeaux-Bacchi, 2011).

Anti-factor H autoantibodies associated with aHUS were first described in 2005 in three pediatric patients (Dragon-Durey et al., 2005). There are several reported cases of anti-factor H autoantibodies in aHUS patients and the literature of this form of aHUS has been reviewed recently (Dragon-Durey et al., 2010a). In addition, the clinical features of factor H-autoantibody-associated aHUS have been described (Dragon-Durey et al., 2010b). This autoimmune form of aHUS affects primarily children but also adults. It often presents together with gastrointestinal symptoms and extrarenal complications, and has a tendency to relapse. Alternative complement pathway activation (decreased C3 and/or factor B levels) at disease onset is frequent in the patients and is associated with a higher risk to relapse and a poor prognosis for renal survival (Dragon-Durey et al., 2010b). It was observed that the autoantibody levels are higher at disease onset than in remission (Dragon-Durey et al., 2010b). In several patients, increase in autoantibody titer correlated with disease recurrence (Dragon-Durey et al., 2010b). Similarly, a patient with persistently high anti-factor H autoantibody titer had several relapses and developed end-stage renal failure (Strobel et al., 2010a). However, in some cases the autoantibody levels spontaneously decrease and the autoantibodies may completely disappear (Moore et al., 2010; Dragon-Durey et al., 2010b).

The presence of autoantibodies to factor H is strongly associated with the deletion of the *CFHR1* gene, which occurs mostly together with the deletion of *CFHR3* (Józsi et al., 2008; Dragon-Durey et al., 2009; Abarrategui-Garrido et al., 2009; Moore et al., 2010). While more than 90% of the autoantibody-positive patients lack *CFHR1*, several of the patients have normal *CFHR1* copy number or at least one *CFHR1* allele. Thus, the decisive factor is the presence of circulating autoantibodies. Therefore, the term previously suggested to describe the anti-factor H autoantibody-associated aHUS, namely DEAP-HUS (deficiency of factor H-related proteins and factor H-autoantibody positive HUS), is not appropriate (Józsi et al., 2008). In addition, some autoantibody-positive patients have mutations in *CFH*, *CD46*, *CFI* and *C3* (Moore et al., 2010), suggesting that a concurrence of susceptibility factors is necessary in some patients for disease manifestation.

The autoantibodies mainly bind to the most C-terminal domains of factor H, i.e. SCRs 19-20 (Józsi et al., 2007b; Moore et al., 2010). Functional analyses showed that the autoantibodies block the factor H-C3b interaction, interfere with the binding of factor H to C3bBb and cause impaired protection of host cells from complement-mediated damage (Dragon-Durey et al., 2005; Józsi et al., 2007b; Strobel et al., 2010a). Most autoantibodies cross-react with CFHR1, because the two C-terminal domains of this protein are almost identical with those of factor H (Moore et al., 2010; Strobel et al., 2011). Immune complexes containing both factor H and CFHR1 can be isolated from patients undergoing plasma therapy (Strobel et al., 2011). Thus, some of the autoantibodies bind CFHR1 instead of factor H, i.e. CFHR1 acts as a decoy, and hence more factor H remains free and functional.

At least some of the autoantibodies show reactivity with other SCRs, e.g., SCRs 8-11 (Józsi et al., 2008) or SCRs 1-4 and SCRs 8-15 (Moore et al., 2010). It needs to be determined whether such autoantibodies affect other factor H functions and possibly the conformation, stability and half-life of factor H in plasma. In some patients, lower than normal factor H levels were reported (Dragon-Durey et al., 2004, 2010b). This should be carefully investigated, also considering the difficulties of factor H determination and the possibility of interference by the autoantibodies with the measurement.

Recently, we have described anti-factor H IgA in three aHUS patients (Strobel et al., 2011). These patients had also anti-factor H IgG and the titer of the IgA isotype autoantibodies were lower than that of the IgG type autoantibodies. Similar to the anti-factor H IgG, the anti-factor H IgA autoantibodies bound to SCRs 19-20 of factor H and cross-reacted with CFHR1 (Strobel et al., 2011). Further studies are needed to determine the prevalence and characteristics of anti-factor H IgA antibodies in aHUS.

Anti-Factor H Autoantibodies in Dense Deposit Disease

DDD is a rare renal disorder characterized by electron-dense deposits in the glomerular basement membrane (Smith et al., 2011). Immunofluorescence analysis shows complement C3 deposition in the glomeruli usually in the absence of immunoglobulins. DDD has a poor prognosis and progresses to end-stage renal disease in half of the cases within 10 years from disease onset. DDD is associated with abnormal fluid-phase alternative pathway regulation as demonstrated by patient cases and animal disease models (Smith et al., 2007). Various autoantibodies have been described in DDD (reviewed in Józsi, 2011). In up to 80% of patients, autoantibodies against the C3bBb C3 convertase, termed C3 nephritic factor, are detected (Schwertz et al., 2001). In addition, autoantibodies to factor B, also binding to the C3 convertase, have been described (Strobel et al., 2010b). Factor H mutations, which result in either quantitative factor H deficiency or impaired regulatory activity of factor H, are identified in some patients (Ault et al., 1997; Dragon-Durey et al., 2004; Licht et al., 2006). In two cases, anti-factor H autoantibodies have been described.

The first described case was a 57-year-old woman who presented with hematuria, proteinuria and hypocomplementemia. Glomerular deposits of C3 and terminal pathway components and intramembraneous-subendothelial dense deposits have been detected by immunofluorescence and electron microscopy, respectively. A lambda light-chain dimer was isolated from the serum and urine of the patient (Meri et al., 1992). This "mini-autoantibody" showed reactivity with factor H and, by binding to SCR3, it inhibited the regulatory function of factor H (Jokiranta et al., 1999). The autoantibody blocked the interaction of factor H with C3b and when added to normal human serum it caused alternative pathway activation by blocking the activity of factor H (Meri et al., 1992).

In the second thoroughly characterized case the patient was a 74-year-old woman presenting with renal failure, proteinuria and hematuria. The patient was diagnosed with DDD. She had monoclonal gammopathy and anti-factor H reactivity. The binding site of the autoantibodies was localized to the N-terminal complement regulatory domains of factor H and factor H-like protein

1 (CFHL1). Functional characterization showed a reduced efficiency of C3b degradation in the presence of patient-derived IgG in a fluid-phase cofactor assay (Nozal et al., 2012).

A recent study investigated the cause of alternative pathway dysregulation in a cohort of 32 patients with biopsy-proven DDD (Zhang et al., 2012). While 78% of the patients were positive for C3 nephritic factor, only one patient had anti-factor H autoantibodies (Zhang et al., 2012). Functional characterization of this autoantibody has not been performed and the binding site on factor H has not been determined.

Apparently, anti-factor H autoantibodies are relatively rare in DDD, affecting only a few patients. In both cases where the antibodies have been characterized in detail, the autoantibodies bound to the regulatory region within factor H and caused impaired complement regulation. It is expected that more cases become known in the coming years as awareness of this form is increasing and detection assays become more available. Systematic studies in large DDD patient cohorts should establish the frequency and the clinical features of anti-factor H autoantibody-associated DDD.

Anti-Factor H Autoantibodies in other Diseases

One case of low-titer anti-factor H autoantibody has been described in a patient with glomerulonephritis with isolated C3 deposits, but has not been further characterized (Sethi et al., 2011).

In addition to kidney disease, anti-factor H IgG autoantibodies have been detected in patients with AMD. In the AMD patient group, both the frequency and the titer of anti-factor H autoantibodies were lower than in the corresponding control group. Furthermore, there was no association between the autoantibodies and the *CFHR1/CFHR3* deletion in AMD patients. The autoantibodies reacted with various parts of factor H, suggesting a polyclonal antibody response (Dhillon et al., 2010). These features are markedly different from that observed in aHUS and DDD patients and suggest that these autoantibodies have no pathological role in AMD.

A study on patients with early-stage non-small cell lung cancer reported that 50% of stage I patients have anti-factor H autoantibodies, 11% of late-stage patients and 8% of the control group (Amornsiripanitch et al., 2010). These numbers are much higher than those reported for aHUS, DDD and

MD. Further studies are needed to confirm this association and describe the characteristics of anti-factor H autoantibodies associated with this type of cancer.

DETECTION OF ANTI-FACTOR H AUTOANTIBODIES

The commonly used method to detect the presence of circulating anti-factor H IgG autoantibodies in serum or plasma samples is enzyme-linked immunosorbent assay (ELISA), as originally described by Dragon-Durey et al. (2005). It is a simple and easy assay that can be performed promptly after disease onset. It is in fact important to identify the presence of autoantibodies as soon as possible in order to adjust the treatment accordingly.

In our laboratory, we measure autoantibodies in serum and plasma samples as follows.

Step 1. MaxiSorp microtiter plates (Nunc) are coated with 5 µg/ml purified factor H (Calbiochem; Merck Biosciences) and control proteins diluted in Dulbecco's PBS (DPBS; Lonza) in 50 µl volume (corresponding to 250 ng factor H per well). The plate is stored at 4°C overnight.

Step 2. The wells are washed thrice with DPBS containing 0.05% Tween-20 (DPBS-Tween).

Step 3. Freshly prepared 3% BSA in DPBS is added (200 µl/well) for 1.5-2 h at 20°C to block non-specific binding sites.

Step 4. The wells are washed thrice with DPBS-Tween.

Step 5. Serum or plasma samples diluted 1:50 in DPBS are added in 50 µl for 1 h at 20°C.

Step 6. The wells are washed five times with DPBS-Tween.

Step 7. Horseradish peroxidase-conjugated anti-human IgG, anti-human IgM or anti-human IgA antibody, diluted 1:1000-1:2000 in DPBS-Tween, are added in 50 µl for 1 h at 20°C.

Step 8. The wells are washed five times with DPBS-Tween.

Step 9. 50 µl tetramethyl-benzidine solution is added. After development of blue color, the reaction is stopped by adding 50 µl 2 N H_2SO_4 (1 mol/l). Absorbance is measured at 450 nm.

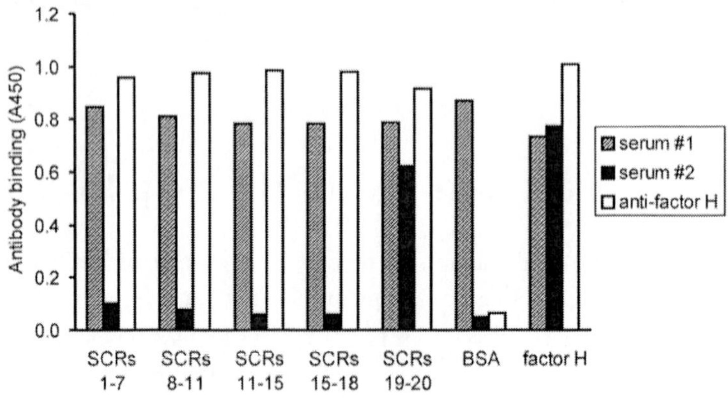

Figure 3. Serum samples are analyzed by ELISA using factor H deletion mutants representing various domains (SCRs) of the protein and also using control protein such as bovine serum albumin (BSA). The figure shows the binding of IgG from a sample (serum #1) for which we consider the binding non-specific and is classified as false positive in the factor H autoantibody ELISA. IgG from serum #2 does not bind to BSA and it binds only to the C-terminal SCRs 19-20 of factor H and is therefore classified as factor H autoantibody positive. A polyclonal anti-factor H antibody is also included as control.

It is important to include appropriate controls, such as bovine serum albumin and other complement proteins (e.g., C3b) as negative controls for factor H, normal human serum samples and known autoantibody positive sample. In our experience, there are samples showing unspecific reactivity to any coated protein and these should not be considered as positive for factor H autoantibodies (Strobel et al., 2010a). Positive samples are further analyzed using recombinant factor H fragments and monoclonal antibodies to factor H, in order to confirm specificity and determine binding sites of the autoantibodies on factor H (**Figure 3**) (Józsi et al., 2007b; Strobel et al., 2010a).

It is useful to determine the antibody titer so that the relative levels of autoantibodies can be monitored during treatment and follow-up to assess the efficacy of the therapy (Strobel et al., 2010a; Dragon-Durey et al., 2010a, 2010b; Roumenina et al., 2011). Rising autoantibody titers may indicate failing treatment and the need to adjust the therapy. Conversely, a declining titer, e.g., due to immunosuppression, may allow successful transplantation (Kwon et al., 2008; Le Quintrec et al., 2009).

Notably, this ELISA measures free circulating antibodies only. It is possible that most autoantibodies are in complex with factor H and the determination of immune complexes is more relevant. It needs to be determined in future studies whether the amounts of immune complexes better correlate with the disease evolution than the amounts of free autoantibodies. Immune complexes can be measured in serum samples by ELISA and visualized in the IgG fraction by Western blot. For the ELISA, we coat various anti-factor H mAbs that bind to different parts of the protein, such as the middle-region and SCR20 (e.g., the mAb C18 [Oppermann et al., 2006]). In samples from autoantibody-positive aHUS patients, the latter antibody detects free factor H only, because of overlapping binding site with the autoantibodies (Józsi et al., 2007b; Strobel et al., 2011). As detection antibody, a polyclonal factor H antibody is used. With this assay it can be analyzed whether the levels of autoantibodies and immune complexes are reduced due to treatment, by comparing samples before and after treatment (Strobel et al., 2011).

Isolated IgG fraction derived from the plasma of the patients can be run on SDS-PAGE and analyzed by Western blot using polyclonal anti-factor H antibody as described (Strobel et al., 2011). This approach revealed that in CFHR1-deficient patients factor H can be detected with Western blot in patient-derived IgG but not in IgG isolated from healthy individuals. Patient-derived IgG isolated after plasma therapy, however, contained both factor H and CFHR1, the latter from the donor plasma, showing the *in vivo* composition of these immune complexes (Strobel et al., 2011).

Importantly, autoantibodies can influence the result of the measurement of factor H concentrations in patient samples. Determination of factor H levels are notoriously difficult due to the fact that the polyclonal anti-factor H antibodies and also most monoclonal antibodies cross-react with other factor H family proteins, such as CFHL1 and CFHR1 (Roumenina et al., 2011; Kopp et al., 2012). Therefore, published plasma factor H concentrations vary greatly. In addition, some of the laboratories calculate factor H concentrations as percent of the level in pooled normal human plasma. Because most aHUS-associated anti-factor H autoantibodies bind to SCR20 of factor H, if in the ELISA a monoclonal antibody is used as capture or detecting antibody that also binds to SCR20, the assay may result in a false low factor H concentration. I suggest that when low factor H levels are measured, this should be confirmed by independent assays using other antibodies for the ELISA and in extreme cases also by Western blot to demonstrate the presence or absence of factor H in plasma.

ARE ANTI-FACTOR H AUTOANTIBODIES PATHOGENIC?

For two of the three published DDD-associated factor H autoantibodies the binding site has been localized to the complement regulatory domains of factor H, and alternative pathway activation and inhibition of factor H function by the autoantibodies *in vitro* have also been demonstrated (Meri et al., 1992; Jokiranta et al., 1999; Nozal et al., 2012). These results and the effective treatment, which led to diminishing anti-factor H autoantibodies, improved kidney function and normalized serum complement levels in a patient (Nozal et al., 2012), strongly suggest a pathogenic role of the autoantibodies.

In aHUS, most analyzed autoantibodies bind to SCRs 19-20 of factor H, which is important for the attachment of factor H to host cells. These are the domains where aHUS-associated factor H mutations also cluster, and these mutants cause impaired control of complement activation at host cell surfaces (Sánchez-Corral et al., 2004; Heinen et al., 2007; Ferreira et al., 2009). Therefore, we have studied the effect of autoantibodies in a host cell protection assay. Human factor H can bind to sheep erythrocytes, which express polyanionic molecules similar to that of human cells, and protect these cells from human complement-mediated lysis. Thus, in normal human plasma sheep erythrocytes are not lysed. In contrast, plasma samples of patients with anti-factor H autoantibodies cause enhanced sheep erythrocyte lysis, indicating impaired protection by factor H (Józsi et al., 2007b; Strobel et al., 2010a). The extent of hemolysis *in vitro* correlated with the autoantibody titer in the analyzed plasma samples. When IgG was removed from the patients' plasma, no lysis occurred any more, indicating that the process eliminated an inhibitor of factor H (Strobel et al., 2010a).

Anti-factor H autoantibodies in healthy individuals have also been described (Moore et al., 2010; Dhillon et al., 2010; Amornsiripanitch et al., 2010). For one such antibody a factor H binding site within SCRs 8-15 was reported (Moore et al., 2010). On the contrary, autoantibodies from elderly control subjects bound to all parts of factor H except to SCRs 8-15 in a different study (Dhillon et al., 2010). It will be important to characterize in detail autoantibodies from control subjects and compare them with anti-factor H autoantibodies from patients to reveal particular features, if any, of disease-associated autoantibodies. Genetic analyses indicate that besides the autoantibodies additional factors ("multiple hit") are necessary in some patients for the disease to clinically manifest (Moore et al., 2010).

Finally, to establish causality and identify direct pathogenic effects of these autoantibodies, studies with purified autoantibodies in animal models will be required.

Relevance of the Autoantibodies to Treatment

Because of the autoimmune nature of anti-factor H autoantibody-associated DDD and aHUS, a corresponding treatment addressing the elimination of antibody-producing cells and, especially in the acute phase, aiming to decrease the autoantibody load is necessary. It is therefore vital that the autoantibodies are detected promptly after admission in order to set the right diagnosis and initiate proper treatment.

One of the two DDD patients with anti-factor H autoantibodies was treated with cyclophosphamide and dexamethasone. Anti-factor H autoantibodies diminished, serum C3 level returned to normal and the kidney function improved (Nozal et al., 2012).

Treatment modalities for several HUS patients with factor H autoantibodies have been reported (Dragon-Durey et al., 2005, 2010b; Józsi et al., 2008; Lee et al., 2009; Abarrategui-Garrido et al., 2009; Le Quintrec et al., 2009; Moore et al., 2010; Strobel et al., 2010a; Boyer et al., 2010). Although many patients have been diagnosed only retrospectively, the available data allow some conclusions. It appears that conservative treatment, fresh frozen plasma infusion, plasmapheresis or plasma exchange are not efficient at long term. On the other hand, data from the literature support a good efficacy of plasma exchange combined with immunosuppressive treatment (Strobel et al., 2010a; Kwon et al., 2008; Dragon-Durey et al., 2010a, 2010b). Some patients received steroids with cyclophosphamide or mycophenolate mofetil, and anti-CD20 (rituximab) was also applied. Future studies need to establish the efficacy of the various immunosuppressive therapies. In addition, the proper diagnosis, treatment and monitoring of autoantibody titers are relevant for those patients who receive kidney transplants (Kwon et al., 2008; Le Quintrec et al., 2009; Dragon-Durey et al., 2010b).

In conclusion, prospective studies need to assess the efficiency of these treatments to establish therapeutic guidelines.

Conclusion

Although the first case of anti-factor H autoantibodies was described 20 years ago, in a patient with glomerulonephritis with characteristics of DDD (Meri et al, 1992), such autoantibodies have received increasing attention only in recent years, mainly due to the discovery of anti-factor H autoantibodies in aHUS patients (Dragon-Durey et al., 2005). Our knowledge on the characteristics of anti-factor H autoantibodies in aHUS has been extended and more cases, also in DDD, are expected to be described in the future. Additional comprehensive analyses of such cases are needed in order to provide more reliable information on the presence and levels of autoantibodies, complement profile, genetic factors, and treatment modalities, which are currently often hampered by the retrospective identification of this autoimmune form. A detailed characterization of the autoantibodies could bring more clarity in certain cases, such as a recently described factor H autoantibody-positive patient developing membranoproliferative glomerulonephritis on the native kidney and the first graft, and aHUS on the second graft (Lorcy et al., 2011). It is useful to determine the autoantibody titer and monitor its changes during disease evolution to assess the efficacy of treatments and allow informed decisions. Further genetic and immunologic studies may identify novel susceptibility factors that predispose to the development of anti-factor H autoantibodies.

Acknowledgments

I sincerely thank all my colleagues who participated in the analyses of anti-factor H autoantibodies in kidney disease, particularly Stefanie Strobel and Harald Seeberger. I thank Barbara Uzonyi for helpful suggestions. The work of the author is supported by grant from the German Research Foundation (Deutsche Forschungsgemeinschaft) Nr. JO 144/1-1.

References

[1] Abarrategui-Garrido, C.; Martínez-Barricarte, R.; López-Trascasa, M.; Rodríguez de Córdoba, S.; Sánchez-Corral, P. Characterization of complement factor H-related (CFHR) proteins in plasma reveals novel

genetic variations of CFHR1 associated with atypical hemolytic uremic syndrome. *Blood* 2009, *114*, 4261-4271.

[2] Amornsiripanitch, N.; Hong, S.; Campa, M.J.; Frank, M.M.; Gottlin, E.B.; Patz, E.F.Jr. Complement factor H autoantibodies are associated with early stage NSCLC. *Clin. Cancer. Res.* 2010, *16*, 3226-3231.

[3] Ault, B.H.; Schmidt, B.Z.; Fowler, N.L.; Kashtan, C.E.; Ahmed, A.E.; Vogt, B.A.; Colten, H.R. Human factor H deficiency. Mutations in framework cysteine residues and block in H protein secretion and intracellular catabolism. *J. Biol. Chem.* 1997, *272*, 25168-25175.

[4] Blackmore, T.K.; Hellwage, J.; Sadlon, T.A.; Higgs, N.; Zipfel, P.F.; Ward, H.M.; Gordon, D.L. Identification of the second heparin-binding domain in human complement factor H. *J. Immunol.* 1998, *160*, 3342-3348.

[5] Boyer, O.; Balzamo, E.; Charbit, M.; Biebuyck-Gougé, N.; Salomon, R.; Dragon-Durey, M.A.; Frémeaux-Bacchi, V.; Niaudet, P. Pulse cyclophosphamide therapy and clinical remission in atypical hemolytic uremic syndrome with anti-complement factor H autoantibodies. *Am. J. Kidney Dis.* 2010, *55*, 923-927.

[6] Clark, S.J.; Perveen, R.; Hakobyan, S.; Morgan, B.P.; Sim, R.B.; Bishop, P.N.; Day, A.J. Impaired binding of the age-related macular degeneration-associated complement factor H 402H allotype to Bruch's membrane in human retina. *J. Biol. Chem.* 2010, *285*, 30192-30202.

[7] Dhillon, B.; Wright, A.F.; Tufail, A.; Pappworth, I.; Hayward, C.; Moore, I.; Strain, L.; Kavanagh, D.; Barlow, P.N.; Herbert, A.P.; *et al.* Complement factor H autoantibodies and age-related macular degeneration. *Invest. Ophthalmol. Vis. Sci.* 2010, *51*, 5858-5863.

[8] Didangelos, A.; Yin, X.; Mandal, K.; Baumert, M.; Jahangiri, M.; Mayr, M. Proteomics characterization of extracellular space components in the human aorta. *Mol. Cell. Proteomics* 2010, *9*, 2048-2062.

[9] Dragon-Durey, M.A.; Frémeaux-Bacchi, V.; Loirat, C.; Blouin, J.; Niaudet, P.; Deschenes, G.; Coppo, P.; Herman Fridman, W.; Weiss, L. Heterozygous and homozygous factor H deficiencies associated with hemolytic uremic syndrome or membranoproliferative glomerulonephritis: report and genetic analysis of 16 cases. *J. Am. Soc. Nephrol.* 2004, *15*, 787-795.

[10] Dragon-Durey, M.A.; Loirat, C.; Cloarec, S.; Macher, M.A.; Blouin, J.; Nivet, H.; Weiss, L.; Fridman, W.H.; Frémeaux-Bacchi, V. Anti-Factor H autoantibodies associated with atypical hemolytic uremic syndrome. *J. Am. Soc. Nephrol.* 2005, *16*, 555-563.

[11] Dragon-Durey, M.A.; Blanc, C.; Marliot, F.; Loirat, C.; Blouin, J.; Sautes-Fridman, C.; Fridman, W.H.; Frémeaux-Bacchi, V. The high frequency of complement factor H related CFHR1 gene deletion is restricted to specific subgroups of patients with atypical haemolytic uraemic syndrome. *J. Med. Genet.* 2009, *46*, 447-450.

[12] Dragon-Durey, M.A.; Blanc, C.; Garnier, A.; Hofer, J.; Sethi, S.K.; Zimmerhackl, L.B. Anti-factor H autoantibody-associated hemolytic uremic syndrome: review of literature of the autoimmune form of HUS. *Semin. Thromb. Hemost.* 2010a, *36*, 633-640.

[13] Dragon-Durey, M.A.; Sethi, S.K.; Bagga, A.; Blanc, C.; Blouin, J.; Ranchin, B.; André, J.L.; Takagi, N.; Cheong, H.I.; Hari, P.; *et al.* Clinical features of anti-factor H autoantibody-associated hemolytic uremic syndrome. *J. Am. Soc. Nephrol.* 2010b, *21*, 2180-2187.

[14] Ferreira, V.P.; Herbert, A.P.; Hocking, H.G.; Barlow, P.N.; Pangburn, M.K. Critical role of the C-terminal domains of factor H in regulating complement activation at cell surfaces. *J. Immunol.* 2006, *177*, 6308-6316.

[15] Ferreira, V.P.; Herbert, A.P.; Cortés, C.; McKee, K.A.; Blaum, B.S.; Esswein, S.T.; Uhrín, D.; Barlow, P.N.; Pangburn, M.K.; Kavanagh, D. The binding of factor H to a complex of physiological polyanions and C3b on cells is impaired in atypical hemolytic uremic syndrome. *J. Immunol.* 2009, *182*, 7009-7018.

[16] Gordon, D.L.; Kaufman, R.M.; Blackmore, T.K.; Kwong, J.; Lublin, D.M. Identification of complement regulatory domains in human factor H. *J. Immunol.* 1995, *155*, 348-356.

[17] Heinen, S.; Józsi, M.; Hartmann, A.; Noris, M.; Remuzzi, G.; Skerka, C.; Zipfel, P.F. Hemolytic uremic syndrome: a factor H mutation (E1172Stop) causes defective complement control at the surface of endothelial cells. *J. Am. Soc. Nephrol.* 2007, *18*, 506-514.

[18] Jokiranta, T.S.; Solomon, A.; Pangburn, M.K.; Zipfel, P.F.; Meri, S. Nephritogenic lambda light chain dimer: a unique human miniautoantibody against complement factor H. *J. Immunol.* 1999, *163*, 4590-4596.

[19] Jokiranta, T.S.; Hellwage, J.; Koistinen, V.; Zipfel, P.F.; Meri, S. Each of the three binding sites on complement factor H interacts with a distinct site on C3b. *J. Biol. Chem.* 2000, *275*, 27657-27662.

[20] Jokiranta, T.S.; Cheng, Z.Z.; Seeberger, H.; Józsi, M.; Heinen, S.; Noris, M.; Remuzzi, G.; Ormsby, R.; Gordon, D.L.; Meri, S.; *et al.* Binding of complement factor H to endothelial cells is mediated by the carboxy-

terminal glycosaminoglycan binding site. *Am. J. Pathol.* 2005, *167*, 1173-1181.

[21] Józsi, M.; Manuelian, T.; Heinen, S.; Oppermann, M.; Zipfel, P.F. Attachment of the soluble complement regulator factor H to cell and tissue surfaces: relevance for pathology. *Histol. Histopathol.* 2004, *19*, 251-258.

[22] Józsi, M.; Oppermann, M.; Lambris, J.D.; Zipfel, P.F. The C-terminus of complement factor H is essential for host cell protection. *Mol. Immunol.* 2007a, *44*, 2697-2706.

[23] Józsi, M.; Strobel, S.; Dahse, H.M.; Liu, W.S.; Hoyer, P.F.; Oppermann, M.; Skerka, C.; Zipfel, P.F. Anti factor H autoantibodies block C-terminal recognition function of factor H in hemolytic uremic syndrome. *Blood* 2007b, *110*, 1516-1518.

[24] Józsi, M.; Licht, C.; Strobel, S.; Zipfel, S.L.; Richter, H.; Heinen, S.; Zipfel, P.F.; Skerka, C. Factor H autoantibodies in atypical hemolytic uremic syndrome correlate with CFHR1/CFHR3 deficiency. *Blood* 2008, *111*, 1512-1514.

[25] Józsi, M.; Zipfel, P.F. Factor H family proteins and human diseases. *Trends Immunol.* 2008, *29*, 380-387.

[26] Józsi, M. Anti-complement autoantibodies in membranoproliferative glomerulonephritis and dense deposit disease. In: Prabhakar S, editor. An Update on Glomerulopathies - Etiology and Pathogenesis. Rijeka: InTech; 2011; 31-46.

[27] Kajander, T.; Lehtinen, M.J.; Hyvärinen, S.; Bhattacharjee, A.; Leung, E.; Isenman, D.E.; Meri, S.; Goldman, A.; Jokiranta, T.S. Dual interaction of factor H with C3d and glycosaminoglycans in host-nonhost discrimination by complement. *Proc. Natl. Acad. Sci. USA* 2011, *108*, 2897-2902.

[28] Kopp, A.; Hebecker, M.; Svobodová, E.; Józsi, M. Factor H: a complement regulator in health and disease, and a mediator of cellular interactions. *Biomolecules* 2012, *2*, 46-75.

[29] Kühn, S.; Skerka, C.; Zipfel, P.F. Mapping of the complement regulatory domains in the human factor H-like protein 1 and in factor H1. *J. Immunol.* 1995, *155*, 5663-5670.

[30] Kühn, S.; Zipfel, P.F. Mapping of the domains required for decay acceleration activity of the human factor H-like protein 1 and factor H. *Eur. J. Immunol.* 1996, *26*, 2383-2387.

[31] Kwon, T.; Dragon-Durey, M.A.; Macher, M.A.; Baudouin, V.; Maisin, A.; Peuchmaur, M.; Fremeaux-Bacchi, V.; Loirat, C. Successful pre-

transplant management of a patient with anti-factor H autoantibodies-associated haemolytic uraemic syndrome. *Nephrol. Dial. Transplant.* 2008, *23*, 2088-2090.

[32] Le Quintrec, M.; Zuber, J.; Noel, L.H.; Thervet, E.; Frémeaux-Bacchi, V.; Niaudet, P.; Fridman, W.H.; Legendre, C.; Dragon-Durey, M.A. Anti-Factor H autoantibodies in a fifth renal transplant recipient with atypical hemolytic and uremic syndrome. *Am. J. Transplant.* 2009, *9*, 1223-1229.

[33] Lee, B.H.; Kwak, S.H.; Shin, J.I.; Lee, S.H.; Choi, H.J.; Kang, H.G.; Ha, I.S.; Lee, J.S.; Dragon-Durey, M.A.; Choi, Y.; Cheong, H.I. Atypical hemolytic uremic syndrome associated with complement factor H autoantibodies and CFHR1/CFHR3 deficiency. *Pediatr. Res.* 2009, *66*, 336-340.

[34] Licht, C.; Heinen, S.; Józsi, M.; Löschmann, I.; Saunders, R.E.; Perkins, S.J.; Waldherr, R.; Skerka, C.; Kirschfink, M.; Hoppe, B.; Zipfel, P.F. Delction of Lys224 in regulatory domain 4 of Factor H reveals a novel pathomechanism for dense deposit disease (MPGN II). *Kidney Int.* 2006, *70*, 42-50.

[35] Loirat, C.; Frémeaux-Bacchi, V. Atypical hemolytic uremic syndrome. *Orphanet J. Rare Dis.* 2011, *6*, 60.

[36] Lorcy, N.; Rioux-Leclercq, N; Lombard, M-L.; Le Pogamp, P.; Vigneau, C. Three kidneys, two diseases, one antibody? *Nephrol. Dial. Transplant.* 2011, *26*, 3811-3813.

[37] Meri, S.; Pangburn, M.K. Discrimination between activators and nonactivators of the alternative pathway of complement: regulation via a sialic acid/polyanion binding site on factor H. *Proc. Natl. Acad. Sci. USA* 1990, *87*, 3982-3986.

[38] Meri, S.; Koistinen, V.; Miettinen, A.; Törnroth, T.; Seppälä, I.J. Activation of the alternative pathway of complement by monoclonal lambda light chains in membranoproliferative glomerulonephritis. *J. Exp. Med.* 1992, *175*, 939-950.

[39] Moore, I.; Strain, L.; Pappworth, I.; Kavanagh, D.; Barlow, P.N.; Herbert, A.P.; Schmidt, C.Q.; Staniforth, S.J.; Holmes, L.V.; Ward, R.; *et al.* Association of factor H autoantibodies with deletions of CFHR1, CFHR3, CFHR4, and with mutations in CFH, CFI, CD46, and C3 in patients with atypical hemolytic uremic syndrome. *Blood* 2010, *115*, 379-387.

[40] Morgan, H.P.; Schmidt, C.Q.; Guariento, M.; Blaum, B.S.; Gillespie, D.; Herbert, A.P.; Kavanagh, D.; Mertens, H.D.; Svergun, D.I.; Johansson,

C.M.; *et al.* Structural basis for engagement by complement factor H of C3b on a self surface. *Nat. Struct. Mol. Biol.* 2011, *18*, 463-470.

[41] Noris, M.; Remuzzi, G. Atypical hemolytic-uremic syndrome. *N. Engl. J. Med.* 2009, *361*, 1676-1687.

[42] Nozal, P.; Strobel, S.; Ibernon, M.; López, D.; Sánchez-Corral, P.; Rodríguez de Córdoba, S.; Józsi, M.; López-Trascasa, M. Anti-factor H antibody affecting factor H cofactor activity in a patient with dense deposit disease. *Clin. Kidney J.* 2012 (in press)

[43] Oppermann, M.; Manuelian, T.; Józsi, M.; Brandt, E.; Jokiranta, T.S.; Heinen, S.; Meri, S.; Skerka, C.; Götze, O.; Zipfel, P.F. The C-terminus of complement regulator Factor H mediates target recognition: evidence for a compact conformation of the native protein. *Clin. Exp. Immunol.* 2006, *144*, 342-352.

[44] Pangburn, M.K.; Schreiber, R.D.; Müller-Eberhard, H.J. Human complement C3b inactivator: isolation, characterization, and demonstration of an absolute requirement for the serum protein beta1H for cleavage of C3b and C4b in solution. *J. Exp. Med.* 1977, *146*, 257-270.

[45] Pangburn, M.K. Host recognition and target differentiation by factor H, a regulator of the alternative pathway of complement. *Immunopharmacology* 2000, *49*, 149-157.

[46] Pangburn, M.K. Cutting edge: localization of the host recognition functions of complement factor H at the carboxyl-terminal: implications for hemolytic uremic syndrome. *J. Immunol.* 2002, *169*, 4702-4706.

[47] Ricklin, D.; Hajishengallis, G.; Yang, K.; Lambris, J.D. Complement: a key system for immune surveillance and homeostasis. *Nat. Immunol.* 2010, *11*, 785-797.

[48] Roumenina, L.T.; Loirat, C.; Dragon-Durey, M.A.; Halbwachs-Mecarelli, L.; Sautes-Fridman, C.; Fremeaux-Bacchi, V. Alternative complement pathway assessment in patients with atypical HUS. *J. Immunol. Methods.* 2011, *365*, 8-26.

[49] Sánchez-Corral, P.; González-Rubio, C.; Rodríguez de Córdoba, S.; López-Trascasa, M. Functional analysis in serum from atypical Hemolytic Uremic Syndrome patients reveals impaired protection of host cells associated with mutations in factor H. *Mol. Immunol.* 2004, *41*, 81-84.

[50] Sethi, S.; Fervenza, F.C.; Zhang, Y.; Nasr, S.H.; Leung, N.; Vrana, J.; Cramer, C.; Nester, C.M.; Smith, R.J. Proliferative glomerulonephritis

secondary to dysfunction of the alternative pathway of complement. *Clin. J. Am. Soc. Nephrol.* 2011, *6*, 1009-1017.

[51] Sharma, A.K.; Pangburn, M.K. Identification of three physically and functionally distinct binding sites for C3b in human complement factor H by deletion mutagenesis. *Proc. Natl. Acad. Sci. USA* 1996, *93*, 10996-11001.

[52] Skerka, C.; Józsi, M.; Zipfel, P.F.; Dragon-Durey, M.A.; Fremeaux-Bacchi, V. Autoantibodies in haemolytic uraemic syndrome (HUS). *Thromb. Haemost.* 2009, *101*, 227-232.

[53] Smith, R.J.; Alexander, J.; Barlow, P.N.; Botto, M.; Cassavant, T.L.; Cook, H.T.; Rodríguez de Córdoba, S.; Hageman, G.S.; Jokiranta, T.S.; Kimberling, W.J.; *et al.* New approaches to the treatment of dense deposit disease. *J. Am. Soc. Nephrol.* 2007, *18*, 2447-2456.

[54] Smith, R.J.; Harris, C.L.; Pickering, M.C. Dense deposit disease. *Mol. Immunol.* 2011, *48*, 1604-1610.

[55] Strobel, S.; Hoyer, P.F.; Mache, C.J.; Sulyok, E.; Liu, W.S.; Richter, H.; Oppermann, M.; Zipfel, P.F.; Józsi, M. Functional analyses indicate a pathogenic role of factor H autoantibodies in atypical haemolytic uraemic syndrome. *Nephrol. Dial. Transplant.* 2010a, *25*, 136-144.

[56] Strobel, S.; Zimmering, M.; Papp, K.; Prechl, J.; Józsi, M. Anti-factor B autoantibody in dense deposit disease. *Mol. Immunol.* 2010b, *47*, 1476-1483.

[57] Strobel, S.; Abarrategui-Garrido, C.; Fariza-Requejo, E.; Seeberger, H.; Sánchez-Corral, P.; Józsi, M. Factor H-related protein 1 neutralizes anti-factor H autoantibodies in autoimmune hemolytic uremic syndrome. *Kidney Int.* 2011, *80*, 397-404.

[58] Schwertz, R.; Rother, U.; Anders, D.; Gretz, N.; Schärer, K.; Kirschfink, M. Complement analysis in children with idiopathic membranoproliferative glomerulonephritis: a long-term follow-up. *Pediatr. Allergy Immunol.* 2001, *12*, 166-172.

[59] Trouw, L.A.; Roos, A.; Daha, M.R. Autoantibodies to complement components. *Mol. Immunol.* 2001, *38*, 199-206.

[60] Trouw, L.A.; Bengtsson, A.A.; Gelderman, K.A.; Dahlbäck, B.; Sturfelt, G.; Blom, A.M. C4b-binding protein and factor H compensate for the loss of membrane-bound complement inhibitors to protect apoptotic cells against excessive complement attack. *J. Biol. Chem.* 2007, *282*, 28540-28548.

[61] Weiler, J.M.; Daha, M.R.; Austen, K.F.; Fearon, D.T. Control of the amplification convertase of complement by the plasma protein beta1H. *Proc. Natl. Acad. Sci. USA* 1976, *73*, 3268-3272.

[62] Whaley, K.; Ruddy, S. Modulation of the alternative complement pathway by beta 1H globulin. *J. Exp. Med.* 1976, *144*, 1147-1163.

[63] Wu, J.; Wu, Y.Q.; Ricklin, D.; Janssen, B.J.; Lambris, J.D.; Gros, P. Structure of complement fragment C3b-factor H and implications for host protection by complement regulators. *Nat. Immunol.* 2009, *10*, 728-733.

[64] Zhang, Y.; Meyer, N.C.; Wang, K.; Nishimura, C.; Frees, K.; Jones, M.; Katz, L.M.; Sethi, S.; Smith, R.J. Causes of Alternative Pathway Dysregulation in Dense Deposit Disease. *Clin. J. Am. Soc. Nephrol.* 2012, *7*, 265-274.

[65] Zipfel, P.F.; Heinen, S.; Józsi, M.; Skerka, C. Complement and diseases: defective alternative pathway control results in kidney and eye diseases. *Mol. Immunol.* 2006, *43*, 97-106.

In: Autoantibodies
Editors: G. E. Jenkins and J. I. Hall
ISBN: 978-1-62081-560-1

Chapter III

AUTOANTIBODIES IN ALZHEIMER'S DISEASE

***Makrina Daniilidou*[1], *Magda Tsolaki*[2], *Thomas Giannakouros*[1] *and Eleni Nikolakaki*[1,*]**

[1]Laboratory of Biochemistry, Department of Chemistry, Aristotle University of Thessaloniki, Thessaloniki, Greece
[2]Third Department of Neurology, Aristotle University, "G. Papanikolaou" Hospital, Thessaloniki, Greece

ABSTRACT

Alzheimer's disease (AD), the most common form of dementia affecting elderly people, is characterized by progressive cognitive decline accompanied by functional impairment, spatiotemporal disorientation and behavioral disturbances. The main histopathological features of the disease include extracellular accumulation of β- amyloid plaques, formation of intracellular neurofibrillary tangles, synaptic loss and neuronal cell death. A growing body of evidence suggests that the "autoimmune hypothesis" may play a critical role to AD pathogenesis. Significant changes both on the number as well as the spectrum of autoantibodies have been observed in the serum and cerebrospinal fluid (CSF) of AD patients, as compared to healthy elderly people. Interestingly, the targets of AD-related autoantibodies are not only neuronal proteins but also non-neuronal antigens displaying various

* E-mail: nikol@chem.auth.gr. Tel: 30-2310-997726. FAX: 30-2310-997689.

cellular activities. In this review we discuss the current knowledge on the nature and role of autoantibodies that have been implicated in the disease onset and/or progression. We further discuss the potential therapeutic approaches based on these findings.

INTRODUCTION

Dementia is a term used to describe various brain disorders with a common characteristic, that is loss of neuronal function. AD is the most prevalent form of sporadic dementia, as it represents 50% of all demented patients. It is a neurodegenerative disorder, currently affecting 5% of the population over 65 years and 20% of people older than 80. It is the fourth leading cause of death in Western societies and more than 13 million people suffer from AD worldwide [1]. AD is characterized by progressive cognitive decline accompanied by functional impairment, spatiotemporal disorientation and behavioral disturbances The major neuropathological features of the disease are the accumulation of Aβ deposits in specific brain regions, the neurofibrillary tangles formed by intracellular aggregation of hyperphosphorylated tau molecules and neuronal cell death [2-4]. AD is characterised as a complex disorder involving genetic background (i.e APOE e4 allele), environmental factors (i.e nutrition) and several pathological conditions (i.e aging vascular diseases) [5]. Many hypotheses regarding the etiopathogenesis of AD have been formulated. The most prevailing is the so-called amyloid cascade hypothesis which suggests a sequence of events triggered by the deregulation of the Amyloid Precursor Protein (APP) metabolism, leading to the production of Aβ plaques, neurofibrillary tangles and finally neuronal loss [2]. Despite the great progress that has been made in the elucidation of the pathways that lead to AD pathogenesis, the whole picture remains rather obscure, as it is very likely that the causes of AD are the resultant of a great number of interconnecting pathological events.

Over the past decade emerging experimental work strongly argues over a contribution of autoimmunity to AD etiopathogenesis. This is mainly confirmed by numerous reports suggesting the presence of autoantibodies targeting neuronal and non-neuronal antigens in the sera of AD patients [6-9]. Furthermore, curative treatment strategies based on active and passive immunization against Aβ peptides have been tested in animal models and in a limiting number of patients with promising results. In this chapter we will discuss the presence of specific autoantibodies in the serum and CSF of patients with AD as well as their use as potential diagnostic biomarkers. The role of the Blood Brain Barrier (BBB) in the penetration of these autoantibodies into the brain parenchyma will also be discussed. Finally, novel therapeutic approaches based on immunotherapy will be revised.

The Blood-Brain-Barrier (BBB): Connection to the AD Autoimmunity Hypothesis

The brain is an immunologically "privileged" region of the body, restricted and protected from the components of the immune system and the antigens. This isolation is consolidated by the presence of the BBB, a structure formed by tight junctions between endothelial cells, a thick endothelial cell basement membrane and astrocytic endfeet [10]. Under normal conditions the BBB blocks the passage of molecules over 400 Da, thus rendering all three major types of immunoglobulins (IgM, IgG, IgA) inaccessible to the brain parenchyma [11,12]. As a consequence the immune system has not developed tolerance mechanisms against brain antigens since B-cells have never been exposed to them [13]. Upon several conditions the BBB integrity may be compromised. This can happen in cases of head trauma, aging vascular diseases (hypertension, stroke, cerebrovascular ischemia, arteriosclerosis) and local inflammation, all of which are risk factors of AD [14,15]. Under these conditions not only the permeability of nutrients and metabolites to the brain is impaired but an excess pass of Igs and other proteins across the BBB occurs. A consequence of this impairment is the anomalous presence of serum proteins in CSF and in the brain. In fact, a deregulation of BBB function is a very common feature in AD patients [15]. There are several reports that document the existence of brain-reactive autoantibodies in serum and Ig bound-neurons in AD cases. [7-9,16,17]. A proposed model by D'Andrea et al. [7] suggests that once a BBB dysfunction occurs, autoantibodies targeting neuronal antigens pass to the brain parenchyma where an amount of them is endocytosed by astrocytes. The remaining pool of Igs is eventually attached to epitopes (autoantigens) in the surface of specific cortical neurons and as a result the neurons become apoptotic. Thus, a prerequisite for the Ig-mediated neuronal and synapse loss in AD pathology is a compromised BBB. This can explain the fact that although brain-specific autoantibodies are present in healthy donors as well, their neurons don't become neurodegenerative because the BBB in most of them, is found intact [7,9,17]. An alternative explanation to the AD autoimmunity hypothesis is that it is the effect, rather than the cause. According to this scenario, the dying neurons are lysed and express stress-related proteins that the Igs bind.

AUTOANTIBODIES AGAINST AB PEPTIDES

Amyloid plaques are formed preferentially by the accumulation of Aβ40 and Aβ42 residue peptides, which are generated by the proteolytic processing of the amyloid precursor protein by specific proteases called secretases [18]. Besides the presence of the insoluble Aβ fibrils in amyloid plaques, several assemblies of Aβ peptides are present in the brain of AD patients, such as soluble Aβ monomers and oligomers. Of these three entities, the oligomers seem to be the most neurotoxic [3,4]. Aβ accumulation in the brain is the result of an imbalance between the production and deposition of Aβ peptides and their clearance from the brain. Pathogenic mutations in the APP, presenilin 1 (PSEN1) and presenilin 2 (PSEN2) genes cause early onset familial Alzheimer's disease (EOFAD) and lead to an overproduction of amyloid deposits [19]. Presenilins are postulated to regulate APP processing through their effects on γ-secrestase [19]. On the other hand, in the predominant form of the disease, sporadic late onset AD, accumulation of Aβ aggregates is generated by an insufficient clearance from the brain [20].

There are several reports that document the existence of naturally occurring anti-Aβ Igs in AD patients as well as in healthy humans [21,22]. Some studies suggest that serum Aβ autoantibodies are elevated in AD and Mild Cognitive Impairment (MCI) subjects, as compared to age-matched controls [23]. These autoantibodies may serve as part of the organism's homeostatic mechanism to clear amyloid deposits [23-25]. Others suggest that Aβ autoantibodies are less abundant in AD patients than those in healthy elderly people and that the reduced levels of autoantibodies to Aβ could be the cause of increased amyloid burden in AD [26-29]. Additional published data suggest that anti-Aβ Igs in human plasma are reactive against oligomeric Ab, but this reactivity descends with age and advancing AD [30]. Furthermore, IgGs targeting amyloid β peptide have been found to decorate the β-amyloid plaques. This is a common feature in AD brains and may contribute to reduced plaque burden in AD individuals [22].

Consequently, Aβ removal via immunotherapy is a prospective treatment strategy for AD. Aβ-binding antibodies of the IgG class can clear Aβ from the brain by the following mechanisms [31,32]: (a) small amounts of peripherally administered IgG cross the blood-brain barrier (BBB) and bind to Aβ peptides in the brain. Microglial cells then phagocytose the immune complexes via an Fcγ-receptor–mediated process that results in Aβ clearance; (b) anti-Aβ IgG bound to the neonatal Fc receptor (FcRn) on the abluminal (brain) side of the BBB acts as a pump to enhance Aβ efflux into the periphery; (c) antibody binding constrains Aβ into a nonaggregable conformation; and (d) according to the "peripheral sink" hypothesis, Aβ binding by antibodies in the periphery disrupts the equilibrium between the diffusible peptide pools on the two sides of the BBB, thereby inducing compensatory Aβ release from the brain. According to this hypothesis, there is no requirement for IgG to enter the brain.

Several therapeutic approaches are currently under consideration, including active/passive immunization against Aβ. In 1999, Schenk and his colleagues [33] made a remarkable discovery, in which administration of Aβ peptide in APP- transgenic mice, could abolish or prevent the cerebral amyloid deposits. Furthermore, two other groups reported that in addition to these effects, active immunization in APP trangenic mice reduced memory loss and improved behavioral symptoms [34,35]. These promising results, obtained in AD mouse models, lead the scientific community to initiate clinical trials by immunizing AD patients with Aβ peptide. Unfortunately, the clinical trials had to be abandoned in Phase II, because 5% of the participants displayed sterile encephalitis accompanied by T-cell cytotoxicity [36]. Passive immunotherapy with anti-Aβ antibodies in APP-transgenic mice, had similar results with active immunotherapy, that is cognitive improvement and decrease in amyloid depositions [37].

Based on these findings novel clinical trials are on the way, using intravenous immune globulin (IVIG) preparations (pooled IgG from the plasma of healthy human donors). Preliminary results, suggest that IVIG administration in AD patients, reduces amyloid plaque formation and improves cognitive function [38]. Additionally, IVIG immunotherapy transiently reduces plasma Aβ peptides and increases serum anti-Aβ antibodies in a dose dependent manner [38]. Thus, it seems that IVIG infusion can mobilize Aβ from the central nervous system into the blood stream. DeMattos and colleagues [39] reported that in APP-trangenic mice treated with monoclonal anti-Aβ antibody, sufficient Aβ peptide clearance was achieved, with no need for the antibodies to enter the brain. These antibodies that were bound to soluble Aβ peptides, reduce Aβ burden from the brain, indirectly, as described by the "peripheral sink" hypothesis. Passive immunotherapy also raises safety concerns, as it has been shown that certain anti-Aβ antibodies (especially those bound to amyloid plaques) delivered in trangenic mice cause microhemorrhages [40,41]. These microbleeds are created by the microglial phagocytosis of the immune complexes. Therefore, antibodies that do not cross the BBB should be free of this untoward effect. IVIG preparations of the IgM class antibodies may also be considered as an option to minimize these side effects due to the large mass of these molecules (900 kDa) as compared to the smaller IgG antibodies (150 kDa). *In vitro* studies, have demonstrated that catalytic IgM preparations from healthy humans inhibited Aβ aggregation, dissolved preformed Aβ fibrils, and supressed the neurotoxicity of Aβ oligomers [42,43]. Furthermore, IgM anti-Aβ antibodies have been shown to reduce cerebral Aβ without crossing the BBB in AD mouse models [21]. Another advantage of the IgM anti-Aβ antibodies is their 2.5 fold higher specific activity against the IgG class. Thus, pooled IgM from human plasma deserves further attention for its use in IVIG immunotherapy against AD.

Autoantibodies against ATP Synthase

ATP synthase is a multisubunit protein complex which catalyzes the phosphorylation of ADP to ATP at the expense of a proton motive force generated by an electron transport chain at the inner membrane of mitochondria. It is highly conserved throughout evolution and comprises of 16 subunits. ATP synthase consists of two domains, a soluble F1 domain and a membrane-bound F0 domain. The F1 component bears the catalytic activity while the F0 component is a proton channel. Interestingly, there are studies that report the existence of ATP synthase at the cell surface of mammalian cells [44,45]. Its location at the cell membrane has been associated with several cellular processes, such as cholesterol homeostasis, endothelial cell survival, and regulation of the intracellular pH [46]. Vacirca et al. [47] demonstrated the presence of anti-ATP synthase autoantibodies in the sera of AD patients. Using an enzyme linked immunosorbent assay, serum anti-ATP synthase autoantibodies were detected in 38% of AD patients, but not in age-matched controls or in patients with Parkinson's disease or atherosclerosis. Additionally, they showed in SHSY-5Y neuronal cells, that ATP synthase autoantibodies could inhibit ATP synthesis, alter mitochondrial homeostasis and induce cell death by apoptosis. The same group also demonstrated that anti-ATP synthase Abs are implicated in cholesterol homeostasis and that they can increase cellular uptake of HDL, a known risk factor of AD [48].

Redox Reactive Autoantibodies

Oxidation-reduction (redox) reactions can "unmask" autoantibody activity in blood and other body fluids from normal, healthy individuals. The agents responsible for this unmasking are molecules that contain transitional metals available for participation in redox reactions. The autoantibodies unmasked by redox reactivities correspond to a growing list of specificities, many of which are responsible for modulating intracellular functions [49]. The evolutionary persistence of this novel autoantibody family indicates that they are important for immunological homeostasis and suggests that they perform necessary physiological functions [49]. AD is characterized by an increase in oxidative stress, leading to oxidation of proteins, lipids and DNA. McIntyre et al. [50] reported a reduction of the levels of redox-reactive autoantibodies and in particular of antiphospholipid antibodies (a-PL) in the CSF of autopsy confirmed AD patients as compared to healthy individuals. They proposed that the decreased a-PL autoantibodies observed in AD subjects could have been previously unmasked by the oxidative conditions in the CNS. These unmasked autoantibodies could eventually gain access to the brain and bind to neurons, leading to neuronal loss [50].

Autoantibodies against Nicotinic Acetylocholine Receptors

The neuronal nicotinic acetylcholine receptors are a family of transmitter-gated ion channels (nAChRs) which contains so far 7 members (α3, α4, α5, α7 β2, β3 and β4). nAChRs are distributed in specific brain regions and are classified in three different binding sites (superhigh, high and low), depending on their binding capacity. They have been shown to be essential for cognitive functions. Low levels of α3, α4 and α7 nAChR subtypes have been found in brains of autopsy confirmed AD subjects and in living patients by positron emission tomography (PET) [51]. Lykhums et al., [52] administered peripherally mice with either recombinant extacellular domains of α4 and α7 subtypes of nAChRs or with anti-α7 antibodies. Active immunization resulted in decreased levels of α4β2- and α7-nAChRs accompanied with an increase of α4β4-nAChRs in brain membranes. Additionally, a decline in episodic memory was observed in mice immunized with α7 domains. Passive immunization resulted in brain nAChR decrease only in mice that were co-injected intraperitoneally with bacterial lipopolysaccharide. The same group further investigated the presence of autoantibodies against the α7 subtype in human subjects. They found anti-α7 antibodies both in the plasma of healthy donors and in AD patients. Among AD subjects they observed an elevation of these autoantibodies in people of 62.5 ± 1.5 years old with moderate or severe AD (15.2 ± 1.3 MMSE scores) as compared to those of 76 ± 1.5 years old with mild AD (22.7 ± 0.1 MMSE scores). These data suggest that the presence of anti-a7 nicotinic acetylcholine receptor specific antibodies are related to memory impairment in early onset AD cases [53].

AUTOANTIBODIES AGAINST GANGLIOSIDE GM1

Gangliosides are sialic acid-containing glycosphingolipids (GSLs) that are expressed in the outer layer of the plasma membrane. They are most abundant in the nervous system, where their expression is cell specific and developmentally regulated. Their quantities and species undergo dramatic changes during cell differentiation and are known to play an important role in neuronal development and regeneration [54]. Yanagisawa et al. [55] found that GM1 ganglioside bound to Aβ1-42, but not to Aβ1-40, form a complex termed "GAβ" in AD brains. GAβ has unique characteristics, including an extremely high aggregation potential and an altered pattern of immunoreactivity, which results in promoting amyloid fibril formation in the brain. More specifically, Aβ binds to membranes containing ganglioside GM1, and upon binding, undergoes a conformational transition from random coil to an ordered structure rich in β-sheet. The formation of GAβ thus provides a mechanism for Aβ fibrillogenesis *in vivo*, therefore serving as one of the critical factors in the development of AD [56]. Chapman et al. [57] examined neuronal degeneration in AD and noted that it was associated with the presence of anti-ganglioside antibodies. A significantly elevated level of antibodies specific to ganglioside GM1, but not to other gangliosides (GD1a, GD1b, GT1b, and GQ1b), was found in patients with AD as compared to age-matched normal controls. In addition, a high level of antibodies to GM1 was also found in patients with multi-infarct dementia and Parkinson's disease with dementia but not in nondemented patients with other neurodegenerative diseases. Another study by Hatzifilippou et al. [58] also revealed elevated levels of autoantibodies against GM1, especially in vascular dementia patients, and this increase was analogous to the severity of dementia.

AUTOANTIBODIES AGAINST OXIDIZED LOW-DENSITY LIPOPROTEIN

Aβ-peptide has been demonstrated to bind with lipoprotein particles in both CSF and plasma and to induce, at high concentrations, oxidation of various biomolecules [59,60]. Indeed, lipoproteins in the cerebrospinal fluid of AD patients have been shown to be prone to oxidation and promote neurotoxicity [61]. Oxidized lipoproteins, and especially oxidized low-density lipoprotein (OxLDL), are also known to be highly immunogenic and to induce systemic antibodies binding to OxLDL [62]. Kankaanpää and colleagues [63] examined the presence of autoantibodies against OxLDL in CSF samples of AD, other types of dementia patients and in age-matched healthy individuals. They determined a significant elevation in anti-OxLDL IgG titers in the CSF of AD subjects as compared to patients with Frontotemporal Lobar Degeneration and controls. As these two diseases represent the most common types of dementia, the usefulness of these findings for the differential diagnosis and disease progression needs to be further investigated.

AUTOANTIBODIES AGAINST SERINE/ARGININE PROTEIN KINASE 1

Recently published data by the authors of this chapter identified serine/arginine protein kinase 1 (SRPK1) as a novel autoantigen in AD [64]. SRPK1 is the prototype and most studied member of the serine/arginine family of kinases and has a leading role in the phosphorylation of SR splicing factors, but is also involved in a series of multiple cellular processes [65]. Interestingly, it has been reported that SRPK1 regulates the alternative splicing of tau protein and in particular exon 10 splicing, which has been involved in the pathogenesis mainly of Frontotemporal Dementia and to a lesser extent in other tauopathies, such as AD [66]. Furthermore, members of the SR family of splicing factors were previously identified as highly conserved autoantigens, especially in apoptotic cells, whose activity is tightly regulated by reversible phosphorylation mediated by SRPK1 [67,68]. SRPK1 itself was also found associated with the autoantigen complex [68].

Autoantibodies targeting SRPK1 were detected in both AD patients and healthy control subjects. A significant increase though, was observed in anti-SRPK1 Abs in the sera of AD cases as compared to age-matched controls. The epitopes recognized by the antibodies were mapped within the first catalytic and the spacer domain of the kinase. Elevated levels of a-SRPK1 antibodies were also detected in AD CSFs but definite conclusions could not be drawn due to the small sample size. According to the authors, aberrant neuronal cell death observed in AD may result in inefficient removal of apoptotic cells. In such a case, SRPK1 that seems to be a major target of caspaces may be released without or with inefficient caspase cleavage thus triggering the initial generation of antibodies. Furthermore, defects in the elimination of apoptotic cell components can lead to secondary necrosis accompanied by the subsequent release of additional intracellular components, like SRPK1, which might potentiate the generation of antibodies [69]. Yet, neither the mechanisms that triggered the production of anti-SRPK1 autoantibodies, nor their potential function and role in the immunopathology of AD have been elucidated. Thus, further investigation will demonstrate their usefulness as biomarkers in the diagnosis and disease progression.

Autoantibody Profiles in Human Sera

In a recent study, Nagele et al. [70] used high-throughput protein microarray technology to identify autoantibodies differentially expressed in 50 AD and 40 non demented control sera. The number of autoantibodies detected was found to be surprisingly high, averaging over one thousand per sample but displaying wide individual variations. A total number of 451 autoantibodies with a significantly higher prevalence in the AD group than in the control group ($p<0.01$) was identified. The authors selected 10 proteins displaying the largest difference between the two groups to serve as possible AD diagnostic biomarkers. Following this approach, AD serum samples were readily distinguished from control sera with a sensitivity of 96.0% and a specificity of 92.5%. AD sera were also distinguishable from sera obtained from patients with Parkinson's disease and breast cancer with accuracies of 86% and 92%, respectively. The presence and function of such a large number of autoantibodies are yet unknown. An underlying hypothesis posed by the authors is that in the case of AD, the somewhat early but selective death of pyramidal neurons provides a chronic source of breakdown products. These products enter the cerebrospinal fluid, diffuse into the blood and lymph, with some presumably acting as antigens to elicit an immune response.

Thus, according to the authors, autoantibody expression profiles, determined using protein microarray technology, can be used to select a relatively small panel of useful autoantibody biomarkers that can detect the presence of AD with great accuracy using only a small sample of blood. Drawbacks of this study were the small sample size and the fact that some of the sera were from living AD patients diagnosed using standard clinical practices. Therefore, this could possibly result in some misdiagnosed cases.

CONCLUSION

Recent acquisitions strongly argue over a contribution of the autoimmune response to AD etiology. The presence of antibodies targeting various specific and non-specific brain autoantigens is a common feature found in AD sera, CSF and brain tissue. While the presence of anti-neuronal autoantibodies in the serum does not regularly lead to any pathological consequence, upon a disfunction of the BBB, due to age-related pathological changes, these autoantibodies pass into the brain parenchyma, where they are allowed to access their targets, thus contributing to the process of neurodegeneration. The opposing scenario suggests that the autoantibodies have neuroprotective and neuroreparative effects and their decreased levels in AD, could lead to the accumulation of amyloid deposits and neuronal loss. Related to their function, the issue of whether the presence of these autoantibodies is a cause or a consequence of disease pathogenesis remains also rather obscure. In any case, their potential use as biomarkers may provide valuable information concerning the disease progression and/or prognosis. Furthermore, increasing knowledge on the nature of the identified AD-related autoantigens will contribute to the better understanding of the molecular mechanisms underlying AD pathogenesis.

Recently acquired data on the involvement of humoral immunity in AD incidence and progression may also provide new therapeutic perspectives. While active immunization against Aβ peptides is now abandoned due to serious side effects, passive immunization seems to be a useful therapeutic strategy. IVIG immunotherapy may prove to be a novel promising therapeutic approach, as it has already been used successfully in several diseases with an autoimmune background.

Acknowledgments

This research has been co-financed by the European Union (European Social Fund - ESF) and Greek national funds through the Operational Program "Education and Lifelong Learning" of the National Strategic Reference Framework (NSRF) - Research Funding Program: Heracleitus II. Investing in knowledge society through the European Social Fund.

References

[1] Ferri, CP; Prince, M; Brayne, C; Brodaty, H; Fratiglioni, L; Ganguli, M; Hall, K; Hasegawa, K; Hendrie, H; Huang, Y; Jorm, A; Mathers, C; Menezes, PR; Rimmer, E; Scazufca, M. Alzheimer's Disease International. Global prevalence of dementia: a Delphi consensus study. *Lancet*, 2005 366, 2112-2117.

[2] Hardy, J; Higgins, GA. Alzheimer's disease: the amyloid cascade hypothesis. *Science*, 1992 256, 184-185.

[3] Selkoe, DJ. Toward a comprehensive theory for Alzheimer's disease. Hypothesis: Alzheimer's disease is caused by the cerebral accumulation and cytotoxicity of amyloid beta-protein. *Ann. NY Acad. Sci.*, 2000 924, 17-25.

[4] Hardy, J. Has the amyloid cascade hypothesis for AD been proved? *Curr. Alzheimer Res.*, 2006 3, 71-73.

[5] Reitz, C; Brayne, C; Mayeux, R. Epidemiology of Alzheimer disease. *Nat. Rev. Neurol.*, 2011 7, 137-152.

[6] Ounanian, A; Guilbert, B; Renversez, JC; Seigneurin, JM; Avrameas, S. Antibodies to viral antigens, xenoantigens, and autoantigens in Alzheimer's disease. *J. Clin. Lab. Anal.*, 1990 4, 367-375.

[7] D'Andrea, MR. Evidence linking neuronal cell death to autoimmunity in Alzheimer's disease. *Brain Res.*, 2003 982, 19-30.

[8] Bouras, C; Riederer, BM; Kövari, E; Hof, PR; Giannakopoulos, P. Humoral immunity in brain aging and Alzheimer's disease. *Brain Res. Brain Res. Rev.*, 2005 48, 477-487.

[9] D'Andrea, MR. Add Alzheimer's disease to the list of autoimmune diseases. *Med. Hypotheses.*, 2005 64, 458-463.

[10] Zlokovic, BV. The blood–brain barrier in health and chronic neurodegenerative disorders. *Neuron*, 2008 57, 178-201.

[11] Pardridge, WM. Blood–brain barrier delivery. *Drug Discov. Today.*, 2007 12, 54-61.

[12] Ohtsuki, S; Terasaki, T. Contribution of carrier-mediated transport systems to the blood–brain barrier as a supporting and protecting interface for the brain; importance for CNS drug discovery and development. *Pharm. Res.*, 2007 24, 1745-1758.

[13] Diamond, B; Huerta, PT; Mina-Osorio, P; Kowal, C; Volpe, BT. Losing your nerves? Maybe it's the antibodies. *Nat. Rev. Immunol.*, 2009 9, 449-456.

[14] Moorandian, AD. Effect of aging on the blood–brain barrier. *Neurobiol. Aging*, 1998 9, 31-39.

[15] Bowman, GL; Kaye, JA; Moore, M; Waichunas, D; Carlson, NE; Quinn, JF. Blood–brain barrier impairment in Alzheimer disease: stability and functional significance. *Neurology*, 2007 68, 1809-1814.

[16] Clifford, PM; Zarrabi, S; Siu, G; Kinsler, KJ; Kosciuk, MC; Venkataraman, V; D'Andrea, MR; Dinsmore, S; Nagele, RG.. Abeta peptides can enter the brain through a defective blood–brain barrier and bind selectively to neurons. *Brain Res.*, 2007 1142, 223-236.

[17] Levin, EC; Acharya, NK; Han, M; Zavareh, SB; Sedeyn, JC; Venkataraman, V; Nagele, RG.. Brain-reactive autoantibodies are nearly ubiquitous in human sera and may be linked to pathology in the context of blood-brain barrier breakdown. *Brain Res.*, 2010 1345, 221-232.

[18] Epis, R; Marcello, E; Gardoni, F; Luca, MD. Alpha, beta-and gamma-secretases in alzheimer's disease. *Front Biosci.*, 2012 4,1126-1150.

[19] Ho, A; Shen, J. Presenilins in synaptic function and disease. *Trends Mol. Med.*, 2011 17, 617-624.

[20] Saido, TC. Alzheimer's disease as proteolytic disorders: anabolism and catabolism of beta-amyloid. *Neurobiol. Aging*, 1998 19, 69-75.

[21] Szabo, P; Relkin, N; Weksler, ME. Natural human antibodies to amyloid beta peptide. *Autoimmun. Rev.*, 2008 7, 415-420.

[22] Kellner, A; Matschke, J; Bernreuther, C; Moch, H; Ferrer, I; Glatzel, M. Autoantibodies against beta-amyloid are common in Alzheimer's disease and help control plaque burden. *Ann. Neurol.*, 2009 65, 24-31.

[23] Storace, D; Cammarata, S; Borghi, R; Sanguineti, R; Giliberto, L; Piccini, A; Pollero, V; Novello, C; Caltagirone, C; Smith, MA; Bossù, P; Perry, G; Odetti, P; Tabaton, M. Elevation of {beta}-amyloid 1-42 autoantibodies in the blood of amnestic patients with mild cognitive impairment. *Arch. Neurol.*, 2010 67, 867-872.

[24] Nath, A; Hall, E; Tuzova, M; Dobbs, M; Jons, M; Anderson, C; Woodward, J; Guo, Z; Fu, W; Kryscio, R; Wekstein, D; Smith, C; Markesbery, WR; Mattson, MP. Autoantibodies to amyloid beta-peptide (Abeta) are increased in Alzheimer's disease patients and Abeta antibodies can enhance Abeta neurotoxicity: implications for disease pathogenesis and vaccine development. *Neuromolecular Med.*, 2003 3, 29-39.

[25] Gustaw, KA; Garrett, MR; Lee, HG; Castellani, RJ; Zagorski, MG; Prakasam, A; Siedlak, SL; Zhu, X; Perry, G; Petersen, RB; Friedland, RP; Smith, MA. Antigen-antibody dissociation in Alzheimer disease: a novel approach to diagnosis. *J. Neurochem.*, 2008 106, 1350-1356.

[26] Du, Y; Dodel, R; Hampel, H; Buerger, K; Lin, S; Eastwood, B; Bales, K; Gao, F; Moeller, HJ; Oertel, W; Farlow, M; Paul, S. Reduced levels of amyloid betapeptide antibody in Alzheimer disease. *Neurology.*, 2001 57, 801-805.

[27] Weksler, ME; Relkin, N; Turkenich, R; LaRusse, S; Zhou, L; Szabo, P. Patients with Alzheimer disease have lower levels of serum anti-amyloid peptide antibodies than healthy elderly individuals. *Exp. Gerontol.*, 2002 37, 943-948.

[28] Moir, RD; Tseitlin, KA; Soscia, S; Hyman, BT; Irizarry, MC; Tanzi, RE. Autoantibodies to redox-modified oligomeric Abeta are attenuated in the plasma of Alzheimer's disease patients. *J. Biol. Chem.*, 2005 280, 17458-17463.

[29] Henkel, AW; Dittrich, PS; Groemer, TW; Lemke, EA; Klingauf, J; Klafki, HW; Lewczuk, P; Esselmann, H; Schwille, P; Kornhuber, J; Wiltfang, J. Immune complexes of auto-antibodies against Abeta 1-42 peptides patrol cerebrospinal fluid of non-Alzheimer's patients. *Mol. Psychiatry.*, 2007 12, 601-610.

[30] Britschgi, M; Olin, CE; Johns, HT; Takeda-Uchimura, Y; LeMieux, MC; Rufibach, K; Rajadas, J; Zhang, H; Tomooka, B; Robinson, WH; Clark, CM; Fagan, AM; Galasko, DR; Holtzman, DM; Jutel, M; Kaye, JA; Lemere, CA; Leszek, J; Li, G; Peskind, ER; Quinn, JF; Yesavage, JA; Ghiso, JA; Wyss-Coray, T. Neuroprotective natural antibodies to assemblies of amyloidogenic peptides decrease with normal aging and advancing Alzheimer's disease. *Proc. Natl. Acad. Sci. USA*, 2009 106, 12145-12150.

[31] Brody, DL; Holtzman, DM. Active and passive immunotherapy for neurodegenerative disorders. *Annu. Rev. Neurosci.*, 2008 31, 175-193.

[32] Paul, S; Planque, S; Nishiyama, Y. Immunological origin and functional properties of catalytic autoantibodies to amyloid beta peptide. *J. Clin. Immunol.*, 2010 30 Suppl. 1, S43-49.

[33] Schenk, D; Barbour, R; Dunn, W; Gordon, G; Grajeda, H; Guido, T; Hu, K; Huang, J; Johnson-Wood, K; Khan, K; Kholodenko, D; Lee, M; Liao, Z; Lieberburg, I; Motter, R; Mutter, L; Soriano, F; Shopp, G; Vasquez, N; Vandevert, C; Walker, S; Wogulis, M; Yednock, T; Games, D; Seubert, P. Immunization with amyloid-beta attenuates Alzheimer-disease-like pathology in the PDAPP mouse. *Nature*, 1999 400, 173-177.

[34] Morgan, D; Diamond, DM; Gottschall, PE; Ugen, KE; Dickey, C; Hardy, J; Duff, K; Jantzen, P; DiCarlo, G; Wilcock, D; Connor, K; Hatcher, J; Hope, C; Gordon, M; Arendash, GW. A beta peptide vaccination prevents memory loss in an animal model of Alzheimer's disease. *Nature*, 2000 408, 982-985.

[35] Janus, C; Pearson, J; McLaurin, J; Mathews, PM; Jiang, Y; Schmidt, SD; Chishti, MA; Horne, P; Heslin, D; French, J; Mount, HT; Nixon, RA; Mercken, M, Bergeron, C; Fraser, PE; St George-Hyslop, P; Westaway, D. A beta peptide immunization reduces behavioural impairment and plaques in a model of Alzheimer's disease. *Nature*, 2000 408, 979-982.

[36] Gilman, S; Koller, M; Black, RS; Jenkins, L; Griffith, SG; Fox, NC; Eisner, L; Kirby, L; Rovira, MB; Forette, F; Orgogozo, JM. AN1792(QS-21)-201 Study Team. Clinical effects of Abeta immunization (AN1792) in patients with AD in an interrupted trial. *Neurology*, 2005 64, 1553-1562.

[37] Bard, F; Cannon, C; Barbour, R; Burke, RL; Games, D; Grajeda, H; Guido, T; Hu, K; Huang, J; Johnson-Wood, K; Khan, K; Kholodenko, D; Lee, M; Lieberburg, I; Motter, R; Nguyen, M; Soriano, F; Vasquez, N; Weiss, K; Welch, B; Seubert, P; Schenk, D; Yednock, T. Peripherally administered antibodies against amyloid betapeptide enter the central nervous system and reduce pathology in a mouse model of Alzheimer disease. *Nat. Med.*, 2000 6, 916-919.

[38] Relkin, NR; Szabo, P; Adamiak, B; Burgut, T; Monthe, C; Lent, RW; Younkin, S; Younkin, L; Schiff, R; Weksler, ME. 18-Month study of intravenous immunoglobulin for treatment of mild Alzheimer's disease. *Neurobiol. Aging*, 2009 30, 1728-1736.

[39] DeMattos, RB; Bales, KR; Cummins, DJ; Paul, SM; Holtzman, DM. Brain to plasma amyloid-beta efflux: a measure of brain amyloid burden in a mouse model of Alzheimer's disease. *Science*, 2002 295, 2264-2267.

[40] Pfeifer, M; Boncristiano, S; Bondolfi, L; Stalder, A; Deller, T; Staufenbiel, M; Mathews, PM; Jucker, M. Cerebral hemorrhage after passive anti-Abeta immunotherapy. *Science*, 2002 298, 1379.

[41] Wilcock, DM; Rojiani, A; Rosenthal, A; Subbarao, S; Freeman, MJ; Gordon, MN; Morgan, D. Passive immunotherapy against Abeta in aged APP-transgenic mice reverses cognitive deficits and depletes parenchymal amyloid deposits in spite of increased vascular amyloid and microhemorrhage. *J. Neuroinflamm.*, 2004 1, 24.

[42] Taguchi, H; Planque, S; Nishiyama, Y; Szabo, P; Weksler, ME; Friedland, RP; Paul, S. Catalytic antibodies to amyloid β peptide in defense against Alzheimer's disease. *Autoimmun. Rev.*, 2008 7, 391-397.

[43] Taguchi, H; Planque, S; Nishiyama, Y; Symersky, J; Boivin, S; Szabo, P; Friedland, RP; Ramsland, PA; Edmundson, AB; Weksler, ME; Paul, S. Autoantibody-catalyzed hydrolysis of amyloid β peptide. *J. Biol. Chem.*, 2008 283, 4714-4722.

[44] Chi, SL; Pizzo, SV. Cell surface F1F0 ATP synthase: a new paradigm? *Ann. Med.*, 2006 38, 429-438.

[45] Kim, BW; Lee, CS; Yi, JS; Lee, JH; Lee, JW; Choo, HJ; Jung, SY; Kim, MS; Lee, SW; Lee, MS; Yoon, G; Ko, YG. Lipid raft proteome reveals that oxidative phosphorylation system is associated with the plasma membrane. *Expert Rev. Proteomics.*, 2010 7, 849-866.

[46] Okuno, D; Iino, R; Noji, H. Rotation and structure of F0F1-ATP synthase. *J. Biochem.*, 2011 149, 655-664.

[47] Vacirca, D; Delunardo, F; Matarrese, P; Colasant, T; Margutti, P; Siracusano, A; Pontecorvo, SL; Capozzi, A; Sorice, M; Francia, A; Malorni, W; Ortona, E. Autoantibodies to the adenosine triphosphate synthase play a pathogenetic role in Alzheimer's disease. *Neurobiol. Aging*, 2012 33,753-766.

[48] Vacirca, D; Barbati, C; Scazzocchio, B; Masella, R; Rosano, G; Malorni, W; Ortona, E. Anti-ATP synthase autoantibodies from patients with Alzheimer's disease reduce extracellular HDL level. *J. Alzheimers Dis.*, 2011 26, 441-445.

[49] McIntyre, JA; Faulk, WP. Redox-reactive autoantibodies: biochemistry, characterization, and specificities. *Clin. Rev. Allergy Immunol.*, 2009 37, 49-54.

[50] McIntyre, JA; Chapman, J; Shavit, E; Hamilton, RL; Dekosky, ST. Redox-reactive autoantibodies in Alzheimer's patients' cerebrospinal fluids: preliminary studies. *Autoimmunity*, 2007 40, 390-396.

[51] Nordberg, A. Nicotinic receptor abnormalities of Alzheimer's disease: therapeutic implications. *Biol. Psychiatry.*, 2001 49, 200-210.

[52] Lykhmus, O; Koval, L; Skok, M; Zouridakis, M; Zisimopoulou, P; Tzartos, S; Tsetlin, V; Granon, S; Changeux, JP; Komisarenko, S; Cloëz-Tayaranie, I. Antibodies against extracellular domains of alpha4 and alpha7 subunits alter the levels of nicotinic receptors in the mouse brain and affect memory: possible relevance to Alzheimer's pathology. *J. Alzheimers Dis.*, 2011 24, 693-704.

[53] Koval, L; Lykhmus, O; Kalashnyk, O; Bachinskaya, N; Kravtsova, G; Soldatkina, M; Zouridakis, M; Stergiou, C; Tzartos, S; Tsetlin, V; Komisarenko, S; Skok, M. The presence and origin of autoantibodies against α4 and α7 nicotinic acetylcholine receptors in the human blood: possible relevance to Alzheimer's pathology. *J. Alzheimers Dis.*, 2011 25,747-761.

[54] Ariga, T; McDonald, MP; Yu, RK. Role of ganglioside metabolism in the pathogenesis of Alzheimer's disease. *J. Lipid Res.*, 2008 49, 1157-1175.

[55] Yanagisawa, K; Odaka, A; Suzuki, N; Ihara, Y. GM1 ganglioside-bound amyloid β-protein (Aβ): a possible form of preamyloid in Alzheimer's disease. *Nat. Med.*, 1995 1, 1062-1066.

[56] Chi, EY; Frey, SL; Lee, KY. Ganglioside G(M1)-mediated amyloid-β fibrillogenesis and membrane disruption. *Biochemistry*, 2007 46, 1913-1924.

[57] Chapman, J; Sela, BA; Wertman, E; Michaelson, DM. Antibodies to ganglioside GM1 in patients with Alzheimer's disease. *Neurosci. Lett.*, 1988 86, 235-240.

[58] Hatzifilippou, E; Koutsouraki, E; Banaki, T; Traka, M; Costa, VG; Baloyannis, SJ. Antibodies against GM1 in demented patients. *Am. J. Alzheimers Dis. Other Demen.*, 2008 23, 274-279.

[59] Biere, AL; Ostaszewski, B; Stimson, ER; Hyman, BT; Maggio, JE; Selkoe, DJ; Amyloid beta-peptide is transported on lipoproteins and albumin in human plasma. *J. Biol. Chem.*, 1996 271, 32916-32922.

[60] Butterfield, DA; Lauderback, CM. Lipid peroxidation and protein oxidation in Alzheimer's disease brain: potential causes and consequences involving amyloid betapeptide-associated free radical oxidative stress. *Free Radic. Biol. Med.*, 2002 32, 1050-1060.

[61] Bassett, CN; Neely, MD; Sidell, KR; Markesbery, WR; Swift, LL; Montine, TJ.; Cerebrospinal fluid lipoproteins are more vulnerable to oxidation in Alzheimer's disease and are neurotoxic when oxidized ex vivo. *Lipids*, 1999 34, 1273-1280.

[62] Salonen, JT; Ylä-Herttuala, S; Yamamoto, R; Butler, S; Korpela, H; Salonen, R; Nyyssönen, K; Palinski, W; Witztum, JL; Autoantibody against oxidised LDL and progression of carotid atherosclerosis. *Lancet*, 1992 339, 883-887.

[63] Kankaanpää, J; Turunen, SP; Moilanen, V; Hörkkö, S; Remes, AM. Cerebrospinal fluid antibodies to oxidized LDL are increased in Alzheimer's disease. *Neurobiol. Dis*, 2009 33, 467-472.

[64] Daniilidou, M; Tsolaki, M; Giannakouros, T; Nikolakaki, E. Detection of elevated antibodies against SR protein kinase 1 in the serum of Alzheimer's disease patients. *J. Neuroimmunol.*, 2011 238, 67-72.

[65] Giannakouros, T; Nikolakaki, E; Mylonis, I; Georgatsou, E. Serine-arginine protein kinases: a small protein kinase family with a large cellular presence. *FEBS J.*, 2011 278, 570-586.

[66] Hartmann, AM; Rujescu, D; Giannakouros, T; Nikolakaki, E; Goedert, M; Mandelkow, EM; Gao, QS; Andreadis, A; Stamm, S. Regulation of alternative splicing of human tau exon 10 by phosphorylation of splicing factors. *Mol. Cell. Neurosci.*, 2001 18, 80-90.

[67] Neugebauer, KM; Merrill, JT; Wener, MH; Lahita, RG; Roth, MB. SR proteins are autoantigens in patients with systemic lupus erythematosus. Importance of phosphoepitopes. *Arthritis Rheum.*, 2000 43,1768-1778.

[68] Kamachi, M; Le, TM; Kim, SJ; Geiger, ME; Anderson, P; Utz, PJ. Human autoimmune sera as molecular probes for the identification of an autoantigen kinase signaling pathway. *J. Exp. Med.*, 2002 196, 1213-1225.

[69] Berg, CP; Stein, GM; Keppeler, H; Gregor, M; Wesselborg, S; Lauber, K; Apoptosis-associated antigens recognized by autoantibodies in patients with the autoimmune liver disease primary biliary cirrhosis. *Apoptosis*, 2008 13, 63-75.

[70] Nagele, E; Han, M; Demarshall, C; Belinka, B; Nagele, R. Diagnosis of Alzheimer's disease based on disease-specific autoantibody profiles in human sera. *PLoS One.*, 2011 6, e23112.

In: Autoantibodies
Editors: G. E. Jenkins and J. I. Hall
ISBN: 978-1-62081-560-1

Chapter IV

AUTOIMMUNITY IN CARDIOVASCULAR DISEASE

Nicholas Parchim and Yang Xia*

Departments of Biochemistry and Molecular Biology and Internal Medicine, The University of Texas–Houston Medical School, Houston, US

ABSTRACT

Autoimmunity is becoming a fairly common issue in healthcare with a clinical syndrome present in up to 8% of the US population. Of all autoimmune conditions, there are more than 80 subtypes that are caused by various autoantibodies against a somatic cell type or tissue. It is the prevailing hypothesis that conditions such as preeclampsia (PE) and cardiomyopathy are the direct cause of autoimmune antibodies directed to receptors within the body. For instance, agonistic autoantibodies activating the angiotensin-1 receptor (AT_1R) and implicated in hypertension, proteinuria, and inhibition of vascular growth. This activating autoantibody (AT_1-AA) plays an integral role in PE. Additionally, earlier studies have shown the role of autoantibodies directed against the β_1-adrenergic receptor (β_1R-AA) in dilated cardiomyopathy and hypertension. The overall impact to patients with autoantibody-induced illnesses can include significant morbidity, concurrent illnesses, or mortality. Overall, these studies implicate the

* E-mail: yang.xia@uth.tmc.edu.

pathophysiologic role of autoantibody in these diseases. Of significance, these findings reveal an earlier diagnostic possibility and autoantibody targeted therapies in the disease treatment.

COMMON ABBREVIATIONS USED IN THIS TEXT

Common abbreviations	
Preeclampsia	PE
Angiotensin-1 receptor	AT_1R
Angiotensin-1 receptor activating antibody	AT_1-AA
β_1-adrenergic receptor	β_1R
β_1-adrenergic receptor activating antibody	β_1R-AA
Muscarinic type 2 receptor	M2R
Muscarinic M2 receptor activating antibody	M2R-AA
DCM	Dilated cardiomyopathy
Soluble fms-like kinase	sFlt-1
Endothelin-1	ET-1
SBP	Systolic blood pressure
DBP	Diastolic blood pressure
IUGR	Intrauterine growth restriction

1.0. DEFINITION OF AUTOIMMUNITY

Healthcare costs are rising steadily and autoantibody-related conditions account for $100 billion in the United States alone. The NIH/NIAID estimates that 23.5 million Americans are affected by an autoimmune illness and the prevalence of such illnesses is rising. [1] It is estimated that 80 types of illnesses have been characterized, but that more certainly exist. Treatment is often difficult due to the varied presentations of illness and causes of disease.

The function of the immune system primarily is to safeguard tissues from foreign invaders and antigens. However, derangements can result in sensitization toward antigens against the body's own intra- and extracellular antigens. Sensitization comprises presentation of an antigen to receptors and activation of somatic immune modulation. It is known that cellular surface antigens and nucleic acids are of significance with regard to systemic autoimmunity via presentation and activation of Toll-like receptors (TLRs). [2] After this presentation, activation of antibody-producing B cells can take place via signaling through TLRs. In this process, a B cell binds an antigen released from an injured cell, internalizes it endosomally, and binds part of it to a TLR. This B cell, in turn, is activated by T cells via a binding of a TLR specific for a self antigen. The B cells can then form plasma cells and secrete self specific antibody and repeat this cycle. Furthermore, mutations in immune-presenting cells can allow for closer presentation between an antigen and B-cell epitope allowing for a greater chance of immunologic reactivity (Figure 1). [3] Moreover, T cells themselves may work to damage somatic organs via suppression of a particular protein that makes one more susceptible to autoimmune maladies. AIRE, or autoimmune regulator gene, controls deletion of self-reactive T-cells.

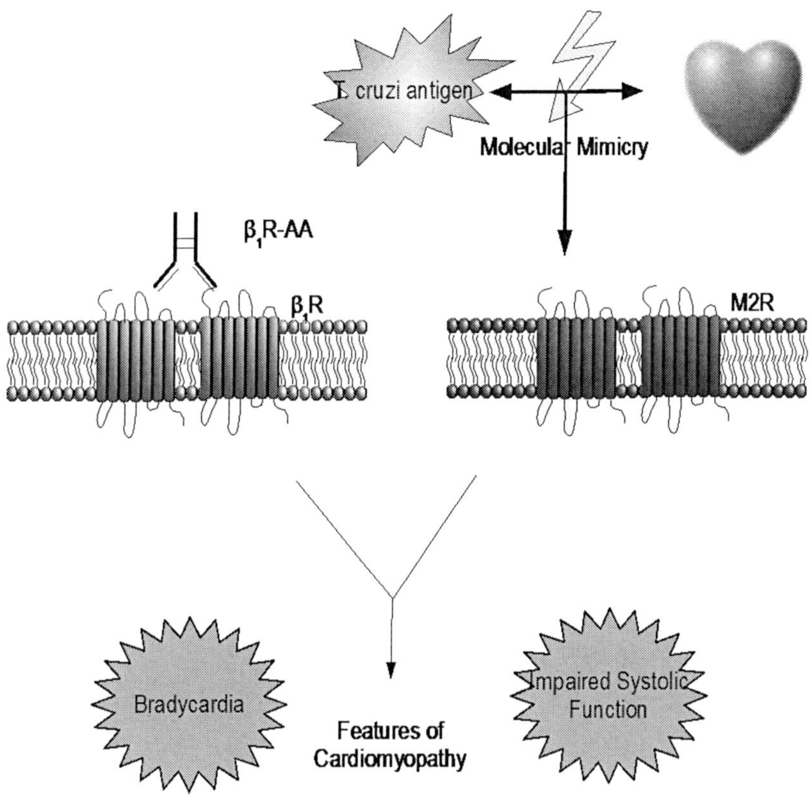

Figure 1. Mechanisms Underlying Dilated Cardiomyopathy. This figure is illustrative of mechanisms that underlie DCM. That stimulation of the β_1R and molecular mimicry stimulation from antigens can form autoantigens to the M2R and cause features of DCM.

Those lacking this gene are more likely to develop autoantibody-related maladies. Selection of these T cells can happen by either active deletion, where T cells produced in the thymus are identified as autoreactive and are deleted, or, by passive deletion where inhibitory cytokines such as IL-10 and TGF-β can inhibit those T cells that are self reactive in the peripheral circulation. Derangement is these processes favors production of autoantibody and could lead to difficulty with deletion of these autoreactive immune bodies. [4]

2.0. Clinical Significance of Dilated Cardiomyopathy and Preeclampsia

As aforementioned, autoantibody appears to play a role in many different conditions. Autoantibodies have been implicated in the pathogenesis of two conditions which have historically been difficult to treat—dilated cardiomyopathy (DCM) and preeclampsia. Symptomatic treatment has been available, but typically does not solve the underlying problem.

Table 1. AHA Classification of Cardiomyopathy

	Classification of cardiomyopathy
Stage	Clinical Definition
A	Patient at risk for heart failure, but no Evidence of structural heart disease
B	Patients with structural disease,without Symptoms of heart failure
C	Patients with past and/or present Symptoms of heart failure
D	Patients with confirmed disease(i.e. Phamacotherapeutic support)

Hunt SA, Abraham WT, Chin MH, et al; American College of Cardiology; American Heart Association Task Force on Practice Guidelines; American College of Chest Physicians; International Society for Heart and Lung Transplantation; Heart Rhythm Society: ACC/AHA 2005 Guideline Update for the Diagnosis and Management of Chronic Heart Failure in the Adult: A report of the American College of Cardiology/American Heart Association Task Force on Practice Guidelines (Writing Committee to Update the 2001 Guidelines for the Evaluation and Management of Heart Failure): Developed in collaboration with the American College of Chest Physicians and the International Society for Heart and Lung Transplantation: Endorsed by the Heart Rhythm Society. Circulation 2005;112:e154-e235.

2.1. Dilated Cardiomyopathy Characteristics and Prevalence

Cardiomyopathy, in general, is defined as any disease of the myocardium which substantially affects cardiac function and stroke volume. Distinguishing dilated cardiomyopathy (DCM) from other types of cardiomyopathy is that the cardiac ejection fraction of the heart must be 40% (normal is defined as ≥ 65%) with an increase in the left ventricular size >115% calculated against age and body surface area. Thus, diagnosis of DCM as is seen today is purely clinical and depends not on serum biomarkers or other factors. For this reason, it is assumed that the prevalence of DCM is greatly underestimated—patients are generally not diagnosed until end stages of the disease course (Table 1). As of 2011, the National Heart, Lung, and Blood Institute estimate that the prevalence of this disease is at least 36-40 per 1,000 population with numbers trending upward. [5, 6]

Even more significant than the statistics about this illness are the treatment options. There are few interventions which can be taken to prevent the disease course from progression to stage D cardiomyopathy.

Table 2. Classification of PE

Classification of preeclampsia			
Classification	Blood Pressure	Proteinuria	Other
Normotensive	<140 SBP and <90 DBP	Negligible or Trace	None
Mild Preeclampsia	>140 SBP or >90 DBP	0.3g Proteinuria per 24 hour period or 1+ Proteinuria on Urine dipstick with 1 repeat confirmation	None
Severe Preeclampsia	>160 SBP and >110 DBP	>5g proteinuria per 24 hour period	Symptoms of maternal Fetal distress, Elevated liver Enzymes, low Urine output, Blurred vision, Headache, IUGR

First line is usually pharmacologic, when symptoms present, in the way of angiotensin converting enzyme inhibitors (ACE-I) or B_1-adrenergic blockers to promote a better systolic ejection. If an infectious etiology is suspected, treatment is usually aimed toward anti-microbials and steroid therapy. However, as stated, since many patients are seen in late disease course, transplant is indicated.

As more is being discovered about this condition and other treatments are investigated, new treatment strategies are emerging. Treatments center around modulating the immune response to repair damage which has already taken place or prevent future damage from occurring. Additionally, biopsy based therapy is becoming common for diagnosis and making a clinical judgment for type of therapy.

2.2. Preeclampsia Characteristics and Prevalence

Preeclampsia is a disease of pregnancy originally characterized by the Greek words "pro" (forth) and "lampo" (shine) meaning to shine forth. This referred to the spots which appeared before the eyes of preeclamptic mothers. In modern clinical terms, preeclampsia is defined as hypertension greater than 140/90 mmHg and proteinuria with excretion greater than 0.3g/24hrs occurring after 20 weeks gestation (Table 2). It is estimated that at least 8% of pregnancies in the US are affected by this condition. It can have serious effects for the mother—kidney damage, abnormal bleeding, headaches, visual disturbances—and for the fetus—intrauterine growth restriction, abnormal placentation and growth, and problems associated with preterm delivery. [7, 8]

With these consequences, it is thought that there would be more treatment options for those with preeclampsia. However, the only definitive treatment is delivery of the baby. This resolves the inflammatory and hypertensive cascade which is presumed to underlie the preeclamptic event. During any pregnancy where a diagnosis of preeclampsia is suspected, close monitoring of mother and fetus is indicated.

In addition, FDA category A and B1 antihypertensive drugs can be given to expectant mothers safely to alleviate some of the symptoms. Nonetheless, decisions to deliver are based on the best judgement of the clinician. If there is considerable risk to fetus and mother, the clinician may decide delivery is in the best interest.

3.0. Dilated Cardiomyopathy Autoantibody Importance

Autoantibody has been implicated as the causative factor in many cases of dilated cardiomyopathy. Unlike other antibody-mediated illnesses, data indicates that there are many potential antibodies involved in the pathogenesis of cardiomyopathy.

3.1. β1-Adrenergic Receptor Agonistic Autoantibody (β1R-AA)

One of the first targets of autoantibody-mediated cardiomyopathy appears to be autoantibody targeting the human β1-adrenergic receptor (β_1R-AA). Initially, the antibodies were found in patients with Chagas (T. cruzi) related cardiomyopathy. [9-11] However, now, the antibody has been linked to depression of left ventricular function and arrhythmia, even in those not exposed to this protozoan. A study by Nikolaev, et al., showed that the β_1R-AA is not present in healthy subjects, but, raised in DCM patients. This leads investigators to show that autoantibody stimulation of the β_1-receptor (β_1R) is functional in DCM. Additionally studies have shown that it is the cyclic AMP upregulation and increased cellular activity is present in cardiomyocytes. [11] Since cardiomyopathy develops over a chronic time course, it would be logical that stimulation of the β_1R could affect contractility, and changes in cardiac rate and rhythm, leading to progressive dysfunction. Indeed, research by Christ, et al., suggested that, initially, the autoantibodies may improve a failing ventricle, however, will soon result in myocyte dysfunction due to sustained contractility. [12] It is the folding pattern of the β_1R in the cellular membrane that influences downstream activity. The pattern of transmembrane helices may favor autoantibody over ligand binding and may modulate receptor conformation and activity.[11]

3.2. Muscarinic M2 Receptor Agonistic Autoantibody (M2R-AA)

The β_1R-AA is not the only autoantibody-receptor combination that has been implicated for DCM. It has long been elucidated that chronotropic modulators have chronic effects on cardiac contractility. Normally, ligands to the muscarinic receptors are responsible for normal basal parasympathetic tone in cardiac tissue. However, autoantibodies to the muscarinic M2 receptors (M2R-AA) display a propensity for pathologic tone. Activation of the receptor results in downregulation of cAMP and increased turnover of phosphatidylinositol turnover. M2R-AA isolated from DCM patient sera showed a stronger affinity for the third extracellular loop of the muscarinic M2R rather than the ligand binding site.[13] This binding of the M2R extracellular loop could have many different effects on the cardiomyocyte due to the duplicitous nature of the receptor.

Stimulation of the M2 receptor has many effects on the intracellular environment. It is hypothesized that stimulation of the third extracellular loop can have partial stimulating and inhibitory effects. Negative effects come mainly from inhibitory effects on L-type calcium channels. This shortens the refractory period and action potential duration. [14] Additonally, a study by Gazinelli, et al. suggests that stimulation of the M2 receptor by autoantibody induces COX-2 and transcription of iNOS mRNA with a subsequent inflammatory response. [15]

3.3. Clinical Significance

Of most significance, however, is the clinical implications that the class of heart problems that the autoantibody can cause. Due to the direct effect on the sinoatrial node, on the major anomalies seen in patients with high titers is bradyarrythmias. This seems to be a direct effect of the stimulation of the parasympathetic tone of the heart.[16] It has been reported that ~75% of those with sinoatrial node dysfunction have an increased titer of this antibody. The influence of the autoantibody is responsible for the bradyarrythmia as well as other arrhythmias, such as atrial fibrillation and ventricular rhythmic anomalies. It is estimated that M2-AA has been present in 25% of idiopathic atrial fibrillation patients and 40% of patients with ventricular rhythm anomalies.[17]

Interestingly, the M2R-AA and the β_1R-AA may have similar, even complimentary effects on the body. As mentioned they appear to be both chronotopic, however, the β_1R-AA affects sympathetic drive while the M2R-AA affects the parasympathetic tone. They are hypothesized to coexist in the same patient but have completely opposing effects.[18] According to current research, it is unclear whether the two antibodies have a net synergistic effect or oppose the other's actions.[19]

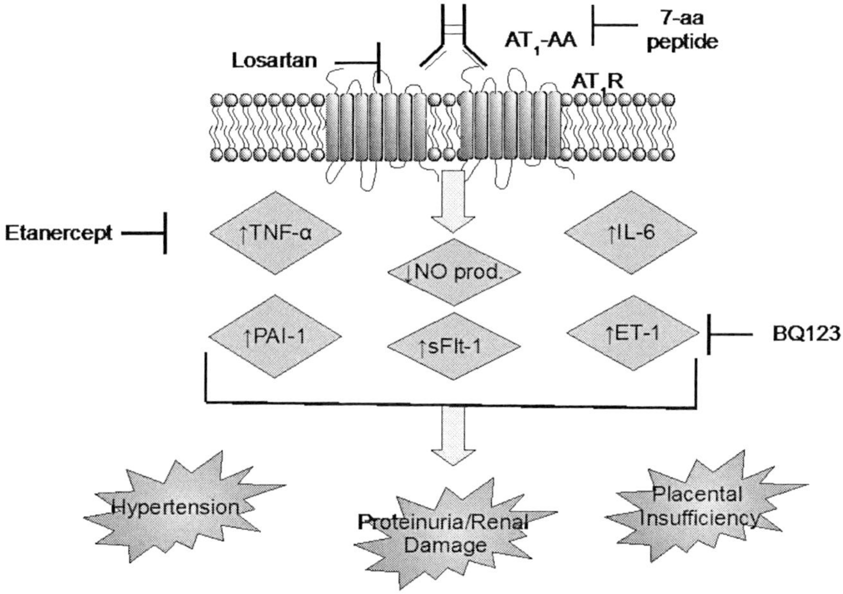

Figure 2. Autoantibody Induction in Pathogenesis of PE. This figure show that by stimulation of the AT_1 receptor, biochemical markers such as TNF-α, IL-6, PAI-1, s-Flt1 and ET-1 can be increased while nitric oxide production decreases. This imbalance leads to the PE features shown, hypertension, proteinuria/renal damage and placental insufficiency.

4.0. Autoantibody and Significance in Preeclampsia

4.1. In Vitro Studies of PE

Even though preeclampsia is identified as a clinical cause of maternal and fetal morbidity, the mechanisms behind the disease remain to be fully refined. The strongest evidence for preeclampsia points to an activating autoantibody against the angiotensin II receptor Type I (AT_1-AA). This autoantibody provides an interesting disease-related and therapeutic topic. Initially discovered in 1999, AT_1-AA was only found in preeclamptic patients' sera but not normotensive pregnant women by using cardiac myocyte contraction bioassay. [20] More recent studies have demonstrated the stimulation of the AT_1 receptor (AT_1R) by AT_1-AA has widespread implications for processes on the molecular, cellular, and tissue level. For example, previous studies demonstrated that AT_1-AA activating AT_1 receptor leads to increases in cytokines TNF-α and IL-6, potent inflammatory mediators and signal molecules. [7, 8, 21-23] Further activation of this system leads to increased plasminogen activator inhibitor (PAI-1), which is shown to be induced in kidney damage and disseminated intravascular coagulation.[24]

Moreover, AT_1-AA stimulation of AT_1 receptor leads to increased PAI-1 production in cultured human trophoblast and subsequent shallow trophoblast invasion, a key feature associated with abnormal placenta seen in PE. Additionally, activation of these factors, in turn, activates NADPH oxidase production in placenta and elevated levels of soluble fms-like kinase-1 (sFlt-1; a soluble vascular endothelial growth factor receptor) and endothelin-1 (ET-1).[23, 25, 26] These factors are responsible for decreased angiogenesis as well as inhibition of vascular relaxation (Figure 2). Altogether, multiple in vitro studies implicate that AT1-AA likely contributes to pathophysiology of PE.

4.2. Effects of PE in Various Laboratory and Clinical Settings

A. Mouse Studies with Adoptive Transfer

As indicated previously, AT_1-AA has the ability to simulate multiple pathogenic factors associated with PE *in vitro.* To test the pathophysiological role of AT1-AA in vivo, Xia laboratory recently have demonstrated that injection of affinity-purified AT_1-AA or total IgG from preeclamptic women into pregnant mice can produce multiple hallmark features of PE (e.g. hypertension and proteinuria/renal damage. Coinjection of losartan, an angiotensin receptor blocker, or 7-amino acid peptide, which binds competitively to the second extracellular loop of the AT_1, significantly reduced AT_1-AA-induced PE features in pregnant mice. In contrast, injection of IgG from normotensive pregnant individuals does not produce the PE features in pregnant mice. Thus, these studies provide the first evidence that PE patients contain a pathogenic autoantibody capable of inducing key features of PE by activating AT_1 receptor. Subsequently, using this autoantibody adoptive transfer model, numerous studies demonstrate that AT_1-AA resulted in the same altered levels of Pai-1, s-Flt1, ET-1 and VEGF that had been seen *in vitro in autoantibody-injected pregnant mice*, confirming earlier findings.[7, 8, 22, 31, 32]

B. Rat Studies with Adoptive Transfer

Interestingly, the correlation between this autoantibody and pathogenesis has been recreated in other modeling beside murine standards. Studies by LaMarca, et al., shows, in rats, compression of the uterine artery can cause inflammatory reactions leading to AT_1-AA production. Moreover, with the compression of the uterine artery, preeclamptic features can be reproduced. Concordantly, levels of TNF-α, sFlt-1, and ET-1 also rose in the serum of pregnant rats. [25, 33] In further studies by the group, the autoantibodies were affinity-purified from serum and administered to day 12 pregnant rats. The injection resulted in PE features including hypertension and renal vascular dysfunction. This is not only significant because it provides an additional model to better study this disease, but also proves that autoantibody production is inflammatory mediated. [34-36]

C. Human Evidence Supporting Autoantibody Role in PE

While this is occurring at a biochemical level, there are changes happening in pregnant mothers on a clinical level. As mentioned, stimulation of the AT1 receptor can lead to hypertension. However, PAI-1, which is a protease important for the conversion of plasminogen to plasmin and formation of clot components. An excess of Pai-1 contributes to kidney damage via extracellular matrix degradation and fibrin deposition in the glomerulus. This can impair the filtration ability of the glomerular apparatus and contribute to the proteinuria and kidney damage seen in preeclampsia.[7] Of additional importance is the derangement in electrolytes within maternal cells. Intracellular Ca^{2+} appears to be increased over normotensive mothers. Thway, et al., has suggested that it is stimulation by AT_1-AA which may be responsible for calcium mobilization especially in maternal platelets and erythrocytes.[37, 38] Finally, studies have investigated the combination of uterine artery Doppler flow and serum biomarkers in combination to predict the chance of PE. While studies have shown that uterine artery flow restriction is an adequate solo predictor of early PE, the combination of uterine Doppler and serum biomarker such as sFlt-1, placental growth factor, pregnancy related plasma protein-A, P-selectin, and neutrophil lipocalin could predict up to 77% of late-onset PE with a false positive rate of 10%.[39, 40] These data show that maternal and fetal changes are occurring on both biochemical and tissue levels. Finally, Siddiqui et al recently demonstrated that greater than 95% of women with PE harbor significantly elevated levels of AT_1-AAs and the level of AT_1-AA activity is proportional to the severity of the disease. [47] In particular, there is a strong correlation of AT_1-AA activity to hypertension, proteinuria and sFlt-1 in severe preeclampsia. Thus, these findings provide compelling evidence that AT_1-AA is highly prevalent in preeclampsia and its titer strongly correlates to the severity of the disease.

5.0. AUTOANTIBODY RECEPTOR BINDING AND PRODUCTION

5.1. Mechanisms Underlying β_1R-AA Production

In addition to autoimmune presentation aforementioned, various other factors can make one predisposed to autoselection of antigens. Research of late has been devoted to whether molecular mimicry—cross-reactivity between a foreign antigen and those of somatic origin--may play a role in pathogenicity. [3] For instance, some correlation has been found between *T. cruzi* infection and antigens and those elciting a dilated cardiomyopathy clinical picture. Interaction with the antigen has some cross-reactivity with sequences within the muscarinic receptor on the heart. [13] Additionally, apoptotic bodies and blebbing from cells may potentiate an immune response from the body. Inadequate clearance from an apoptotic cell may result in presentation of antigens from within the cell to TLRs and, thus, production of lymphocytes. [41, 42]

5.2. Mechanisms Underlying AT_1-AA Production and Function

One of the prevailing theories underlying autoantibody production is insult resulting in sensitization to self antigens. In their previous rat studies, LaMarca, et al., have shown that hypoxia via clamping of the uterine artery results in an inflammatory condition that could increase production of autoantibody.[25, 33, 36, 43] Indeed, this could be resultant from cellular damage, whereby cellular contents are extruded and presented to B cells. This restricted uterine perfusion model showed that the hypoxic insult is required to start the generation of autoantibody and continue the cascade of damage. While this does not address why some patients are more likely to develop PE than others, it provides an explanation for presentation of self antigens.

Also of note is the question of how AT_1-AA actually is active on the receptor. It is known that the AT_1 receptor is G-protein linked for intracellular signaling. It was previously thought that G-protein couple receptor (GPCR) complexes were just monomers. It is now known that GPCRs can dimerize and form complexes with one G protein complex. AbdAlla, et al., have shown that dimerization is necessary for activation and responsiveness in the AT_1 receptor. [38] Blocking dimerization could reduce the singnalling potential of the receptor. This is important since it implies a therapeutic potential for this receptor mediated disease.

6.0. THERAPEUTIC CONSIDERATIONS

6.1. Dilated Cardiomyopathic Treatment

While there is no accepted treatment for DCM, there have been many options considered for abatement. In the case of DCM, one of the main targets has been the blockade of the β_1-adrenergic receptor. However, the block is only partial—carvedilol (a β_1 blocker) could only block 60-70% of cAMP activity at maximum. This beta-blocker treatment is also a mainstay of DCM treatment in general, and not for abolition of the condition. Other approaches are currently examining targeting the autoantibodies to the β_1-receptor by immunoadsorption or by targeting antibody-producing B-cells themselves. [11]

The M2R might be a further target for modulation of DCM. It is hypothesized that there are two significant approaches which may work. Studies have shown that infusion of M2 receptor peptide was found to improve contractility of the heart and mitigate inflammation.[15] Furthermore, as with many autoantibody mediated illnesses, infusion of intravenous immunoglobulin has been shown to be palliative. The infusion of this immunoglobulin appears to have actions against the Fc-receptor activity. [44]

6.2. Preeclampsia Treatment

While the symptomatic treatment for PE has been well studied, it appears that the curative treatment for PE is more obscure. Success has been found *in vitro* and partially *in vivo* with the administration of Losartan, an angiotensin receptor blocker, and 7-amino acid peptide, which binds competitively to the second extracellular loop of the AT_1R. Currently, these treatments are not FDA approved, however, the ablation strategy used in these therapies is valuable for future research and therapeutic targeting. As aforementioned, TNF-α has been implicated as a very important cytokine and signaling molecule for PE. Some studies have found that administration of a TNF-α blocker, Etanercept, can partially abrogate some of the features of PE, providing another valuable therapeutic target.[43, 45]

More interestingly, several new strategies are looking at further targets within the PE pathway. Extensive work by LaMarca BB and JP Granger lead to another therapeutic target with ET-1 and the receptor ET_a. Work in their laboratory has shown ET-1 to be important for invasion of the trophoblast and pivotal role in hypertension allowing the discussion that it be a therapeutic target.[25, 33, 43, 46] Work by Zhou, et al. also confirmed this that abatement and inhibition of IL-6 and ET-1 can prove to reduce preeclamptic features in mice.[26] Their research showed that with an inhibitor of ET-1, BQ123, This type of target could easily be translated to human trials.

Conclusion

As autoantibody research brings to the forefront many new conditions, there may be a shift in accepted treatment strategies for many conditions. Already, clinical medicine is beginning to look to immunologic mechanisms underlying disorders to find new treatment protocols. Within the next decades, where there were previously no accepted treatments for autoimmune diseases, including DCM and PE, there may be new strategies that are curative rather than palliative. However, this is purely dependent on researching mechanistically rather than looking at individual symptomology.

References

[1] NIAID Autoimmune Diseases. *Selected Scientific Areas of Research*, 52-53.

[2] Green, N.M. and A. Marshak-Rothstein, Toll-like receptor driven B cell activation in the induction of systemic autoimmunity. *Semin. Immunol.*, 2011. 23(2): p. 106-12.

[3] Racanelli, V., et al., Autoantibodies to intracellular antigens: generation and pathogenetic role. *Autoimmun. Rev.*, 2011. 10(8): p. 503-8.

[4] Murphy, K., P. Travers, M. Walport, *Janeway's Immunobiology*. 2008, Garland Science: New York. p. 607-619.

[5] Bott-Silverman, C. (2011) Dilated and Restrictive Cardiomyopathies. *Disease Management Project.*

[6] Heinz-Peter Schultheiss, U.K., Drugs and/or devices in dilated cardiomyopathy. *Heart and Metabolism*, 2011(49): p. 9-12.

[7] Irani, R.A. and Y. Xia, The functional role of the renin-angiotensin system in pregnancy and preeclampsia. *Placenta*, 2008. 29(9): p. 763-71.

[8] Irani, R.A. and Y. Xia, Renin angiotensin signaling in normal pregnancy and preeclampsia. *Semin. Nephrol.,* 2011. 31(1): p. 47-58.

[9] Borda, E., et al., A circulating IgG in Chagas' disease which binds to beta-adrenoceptors of myocardium and modulates their activity. *Clin. Exp. Immunol.,* 1984. 57(3): p. 679-86.

[10] Elies, R., et al., Structural and functional analysis of the B cell epitopes recognized by anti-receptor autoantibodies in patients with Chagas' disease. *J. Immunol.*, 1996. 157(9): p. 4203-11.

[11] Nikolaev, V.O., et al., A novel fluorescence method for the rapid detection of functional beta1-adrenergic receptor autoantibodies in heart failure. *J. Am. Coll. Cardiol.,* 2007. 50(5): p. 423-31.

[12] Christ, T., et al., Autoantibodies against the beta1 adrenoceptor from patients with dilated cardiomyopathy prolong action potential duration and enhance contractility in isolated cardiomyocytes. *J. Mol. Cell. Cardiol., 2001. 33(8): p. 1515-25.*

[13] Nussinovitch, U. and Y. Shoenfeld, The Diagnostic and Clinical Significance of Anti-Muscarinic Receptor Autoantibodies. *Clin. Rev. Allergy Immunol., 2011.*

[14] Nascimento, J.H., et al., cGMP-mediated inhibition of cardiac L-type Ca(2+) current by a monoclonal antibody against the M(2) ACh receptor. *Am. J. Physiol. Cell. Physiol., 2001.* 281(4): p. C1251-8.

[15] Ganzinelli, S., et al., Chagasic antibodies induce cardiac COX-2/iNOS mRNA expression with PGE2/NO production. *Int. J. Cardiol.*, 2009. 134(2): p. 212-23.

[16] Baba, A., et al., Autoantibodies against M2-muscarinic acetylcholine receptors: new upstream targets in atrial fibrillation in patients with dilated cardiomyopathy. *Eur. Heart J.,* 2004. 25(13): p. 1108-15.

[17] Lazzerini, P.E., et al., Autoantibody-mediated cardiac arrhythmias: mechanisms and clinical implications. *Basic Res. Cardiol.*, 2008. 103(1): p. 1-11.

[18] Matsui, S., et al., Transfer of immune components from rabbit autoimmune cardiomyopathy into severe combined immunodeficiency (SCID) mice induces cardiomyopathic changes. *Autoimmunity*, 2006. 39(2): p. 121-8.

[19] Peter, J.C., et al., Effects on heart rate of an anti-M2 acetylcholine receptor immune response in mice. *FASEB J.,* 2005. 19(8): p. 943-9.

[20] Wallukat, G., et al., Patients with preeclampsia develop agonistic autoantibodies against the angiotensin AT1 receptor. *J. Clin. Invest.,* 1999. 103(7): p. 945-52.

[21] Irani, R.A., et al., Autoantibody-mediated angiotensin receptor activation contributes to preeclampsia through tumor necrosis factor-alpha signaling. *Hypertension*, 2010. 55(5): p. 1246-53.

[22] Zhou, C.C., et al., Autoantibody-mediated IL-6-dependent endothelin-1 elevation underlies pathogenesis in a mouse model of preeclampsia. *J. Immunol.*, 2011. 186(10): p. 6024-34.

[23] Xia, Y. and R.E. Kellems, Receptor-activating autoantibodies and disease: preeclampsia and beyond. *Expert Rev. Clin. Immunol.*, 2011. 7(5): p. 659-74.

[24] Bobst, S.M., et al., Maternal autoantibodies from preeclamptic patients activate angiotensin receptors on human mesangial cells and induce interleukin-6 and plasminogen activator inhibitor-1 secretion. *Am. J. Hypertens,* 2005. 18(3): p. 330-6.

[25] LaMarca, B., et al., Hypertension in response to autoantibodies to the angiotensin II type I receptor (AT1-AA) in pregnant rats: role of endothelin-1. *Hypertension,* 2009. 54(4): p. 905-9.

[26] Siddiqui, A.H., et al., Angiotensin receptor agonistic autoantibody is highly prevalent in preeclampsia: correlation with disease severity. *Hypertension*, 2010. 55(2): p. 386-93.

[27] de Oliveira, L.G., A. Karumanchi, and N. Sass, [Preeclampsia: oxidative stress, inflammation and endothelial dysfunction]. *Rev. Bras. Ginecol. Obstet*, 2010. 32(12): p. 609-16.

[28] Khankin, E.V., et al., Hemodynamic, Vascular, and Reproductive Impact of FMS-Like Tyrosine Kinase 1 (FLT1) Blockade on the Uteroplacental Circulation During Normal Mouse Pregnancy. *Biol. Reprod.*, 2011.

[29] Agarwal, I. and S.A. Karumanchi, Preeclampsia and the Anti-Angiogenic State. *Pregnancy Hypertens*, 2011. 1(1): p. 17-21.

[30] Li, F., et al., eNOS Deficiency Acts through Endothelin to Aggravate sFlt-1-Induced Pre-Eclampsia-Like Phenotype. *J. Am. Soc. Nephrol.*, 2012.

[31] Zhou, C.C., et al., Angiotensin receptor agonistic autoantibodies induce pre-eclampsia in pregnant mice. *Nat. Med.*, 2008. 14(8): p. 855-62.
[32] Irani, R.A., et al., The detrimental role of angiotensin receptor agonistic autoantibodies in intrauterine growth restriction seen in preeclampsia. *J. Exp. Med.*, 2009. 206(12): p. 2809-22.
[33] LaMarca, B., et al., Autoantibodies to the angiotensin type I receptor in response to placental ischemia and tumor necrosis factor alpha in pregnant rats. *Hypertension*, 2008. 52(6): p. 1168-72.
[34] Parrish, M.R., et al., The effect of immune factors, tumor necrosis factor-alpha, and agonistic autoantibodies to the angiotensin II type I receptor on soluble fms-like tyrosine-1 and soluble endoglin production in response to hypertension during pregnancy. *Am. J. Hypertens.*, 2010. 23(8): p. 911-6.
[35] Parrish, M.R., et al., Angiotensin II type 1 autoantibody induced hypertension during pregnancy is associated with renal endothelial dysfunction. *Gend. Med.*, 2011. 8(3): p. 184-8.
[36] Parrish, M.R., et al., Hypertension in response to AT1-AA: role of reactive oxygen species in pregnancy-induced hypertension. *Am. J. Hypertens.*, 2011. 24(7): p. 835-40.
[37] Haller, H., et al., Increased intracellular free calcium and sensitivity to angiotensin II in platelets of preeclamptic women. *Am. J. Hypertens.*, 1989. 2(4): p. 238-43.
[38] AbdAlla, S., H. Lother, and U. Quitterer, AT1-receptor heterodimers show enhanced G-protein activation and altered receptor sequestration. *Nature*, 2000. 407(6800): p. 94-8.
[39] Ghosh, S.K., et al., Combination of uterine artery Doppler velocimetry and maternal serum placental growth factor estimation in predicting occurrence of pre-eclampsia in early second trimester pregnancy: a prospective cohort study. *Eur. J. Obstet. Gynecol. Reprod. Biol.,* 2012.
[40] Youssef, A., et al., Uterine artery Doppler and biochemical markers (PAPP-A, PIGF, sFlt-1, P-selectin, NGAL) at 11 + 0 to 13 + 6 weeks in the prediction of late (> 34 weeks) pre-eclampsia. *Prenat Diagn*, 2011. 31(12): p. 1141-6.
[41] Fransen, J.H., et al., Mouse dendritic cells matured by ingestion of apoptotic blebs induce T cells to produce interleukin-17. *Arthritis. Rheum.,* 2009. 60(8): p. 2304-13.
[42] Fehr, E.M., et al., Apototic cell-derived membrane vesicles induce CD83 expression on human mdDC. *Autoimmunity*, 2009. 42(4): p. 322-4.

[43] LaMarca, B.B., et al., Role of endothelin in mediating tumor necrosis factor-induced hypertension in pregnant rats. *Hypertension*, 2005. 46(1): p. 82-6.

[44] Nussinovitch, U. and Y. Shoenfeld, Intravenous immunoglobulin - indications and mechanisms in cardiovascular diseases. *Autoimmun. Rev.*, 2008. 7(6): p. 445-52.

[45] Marsden, P.A. and B.M. Brenner, Transcriptional regulation of the endothelin-1 gene by TNF-alpha. *Am. J. Physiol.*, 1992. 262(4 Pt 1): p. C854-61.

[46] George, E.M. and J.P. Granger, Endothelin: key mediator of hypertension in preeclampsia. *Am. J. Hypertens.*, 2011. 24(9): p. 964-9.

[47] Siddiqui, A. H., R. A. Irani, Y. Zhang, Y. Dai, S. C. Blackwell, S. M. Ramin, R. E. Kellems, and Y. Xia. Recombinant Vascular Endothelial Growth Factor 121 Attenuates Autoantibody-induced Features of Pre-eclampsia in Pregnant Mice. *Am. J. Hypertens*. 24.5 (2011): 606-12.

In: Autoantibodies
Editors: G. E. Jenkins and J. I. Hall
ISBN: 978-1-62081-560-1

Chapter V

APPROACHES FOR DETECTION AND ANALYSIS OF NATURAL AUTOANTIBODIES

***Naohito Nishii*[1] *and Hitoshi Kitagawa*[2]**
[1] Laboratory of Veterinary Pharmacotherapeutics, Faculty of Agriculture, Tottori University, Japan
[2] Laboratory of Veterinary Internal Medicine, Faculty of Applied Biological Sciences, Gifu University, Japan

ABSTRACT

A normal immune system contains autoantibodies against self-antigens, termed as termed natural autoantibodies (NAAbs). NAAbs are found in many species, and appear to be conserved through evolution. The physiological significance of NAAbs is not well understood; however, it is postulated that NAAbs have various biological roles, such as first line protection against infection, immunoregulation, and clearance of altered self antigens.

Recently, we have detected NAAbs against insulin in healthy cats while developing an enzyme-linked immunosorbent assay (ELISA) for determining feline serum insulin concentration. Our study showed that feline NAAbs against insulin were polyclonal/polyreactive and had a high affinity and binding capacity. In this review, we outline the nature of NAAbs and the methods for detecting and analyzing of NAAbs, including ELISA for screening, affinity chromatography, competitive radioimmunoassay, and epitope analysis.

INTRODUCTION

Natural autoantibodies (NAAbs) are autoantibodies observed in healthy individuals. NAAbs have been investigated for over three decades, and researchers have tried to analyze them using various tactics. Assays for antibodies are normally used for detecting autoantibodies in patients with autoimmune diseases. In these assays, NAAbs are treated as a background binding. To detect and analyze the NAAbs, a more sensitive technique is required, as NAAbs tend to have low-affinity. The aim of this review is to summarize the characteristics of NAAbs and to cite a case of detection and analysis of NAAbs.

IMMUNE TOLERANCE AND NATURAL AUTOANTIBODIES

A healthy immune system has the ability to remove self-reacting B cells. The acquisition of self-tolerance in B cells is achieved during cell development. In the bone marrow, B cells that have high avidity to self antigens receive receptor editing, which modifies the B cell receptor making it non-reactive. After receptor editing, the B cells that still have autoreactivity are removed apoptosis. This process for development of B cell tolerance is termed "central tolerance." However, some self antigens are expressed specifically in peripheral organs and not in the bone marrow. Thus, B cells that react with these peripheral antigens emigrate to the periphery. The immune system depletes such peripheral antigen-reacting B cells through a process called "peripheral tolerance." In this process, self-reactive B cells are deleted or anergized.

Autoantibodies are antibodies that react with autoantigens; thus, the generation of autoantibodies is a consequence of a defect in self-tolerance toward autoantigens. Autoantibodies are generally recognized as pathogenic because high titers of autoantigens have been detected in patients with various autoimmune diseases. Therefore, the presence of autoantibodies was considered synonymous with autoimmune diseases [13]. However, evidence has shown that autoantibodies exist in the blood of healthy individuals. These antibodies bind to self antigens and are termed as "natural autoantibodies (NAAbs)." NAAbs are known to react with various self antigens, such as single-stranded DNA, immunoglobulins, cell surface molecules, and cytokines [5, 9, 10]. Although B cells with self-reactivity are deleted or their reactivity is modified in the course of development, this process is not flawless. In fact, B cells are positively selected via binding to self antigens [10]. Thus, it can be said that a certain amount of NAAbs is present in the blood of healthy individuals.

"Natural antibodies" are known to exist intrinsically without any pathogenic stimulation. Many natural antibodies can bind with self antigens, therefore NAAbs are a part of natural antibodies. It is important to understand the difference between these two terms, which are based on different concepts.

CHARACTERISTICS OF NATURAL AUTOANTIBODIES

NAAbs are produced mainly by B-1 cells, which are enriched in the peritoneal and pleural cavities [19]. B-1 cells are further subdivided into CD5+ B-1a and CD5- B-1b cells [22]. Although B-1 cells have recently become a focus of intense study, their properties and biological roles still remain unclear.

NAAbs comprise IgM, IgG, and IgA. Initial studies show that NAAbs are predominantly IgM because NAAbs from the serum of newborn mice exclusively contained IgM [12]. However, this were true only in newborn or germ-free individuals, as most of the NAAbs in the serum of adult individuals are found to be IgG [1]. We also reported autoreactive IgG antibodies are present in healthy adult cats [17].

The repertoire of NAAbs detected in the neonate or cord blood is restricted to a limited set of self antigens and is highly conserved among individuals [12]. This observation is consistent with the fact that B cells undergo positive selection by self antigens, as mentioned previously. The repertoire of autoreactive IgM increases in diversity within the first 2 years of life, which could be because of stimulation by external antigens. Self-reactive IgG is also produced during this period. The established repertoire of NAAbs against self antigens is conserved among individuals and does not change drastically throughout the lifespan [15], although the repertoire of NAAbs toward external antigens is highly diverse [11].

Most NAAbs are polyclonal/polyreactive, although monoclonal NAAbs have also been reported [12]. The polyreactivity is toward not only self antigens but also external antigens. This reactivity toward external antigens such as pathogens acts as an immunological defense.

Biological Role of Natural Autoantibodies

Although the biological role of NAAbs is yet to be investigated, several hypotheses have been suggested. First, NAAbs are known to bind to various pathogens, thereby acting as the first line of immunological defense [13, 22]. Pathogens bound with antibodies are then lysed by a complement system or neutralized. For example, pre-existing natural antibodies ameliorate disease outcome following influenza virus infection in mice, and the lack of natural antibodies causes severe consequences during overwhelming sepsis and other infections [4]. Of note, infection of influenza virus did not increase the level of natural antibodies that bind to the virus [3]. Furthermore, immunoregulation by NAAbs has been reported. Immunoregulation is performed through idiotypic interactions, modulation of cytokine action, and interaction with T and B cells [2]. These effects might prevent individuals from pathogenesis of autoimmune diseases. NAAbs are also suspected tobe involved in the induction of autoimmune disease [20]. In addition, NAAbs have an important role in the scavenging action for senescent or altered molecules, cells, or tumors [6]. For example, the in vitro phagocytosis of erythrocytes is related to the binding of natural anti-Gal antibodies, which suggests that the removal of senescent erythrocytes is accelerated by NAAbs [7].

NAAbs react with self antigens that are also targets for autoantibodies in autoimmune disease [12]. However, the mechanisms that protect NAAbs from the induction of autoimmune disease are not well known. Concerning this crucial issue, several lines of evidence have been reported. Compared with healthy individuals, the NAAb titer was found to be significantly high in individuals with autoimmune diseased, and the target epitope differed between the two groups [1, 14, 16, 21]. In addition, anti-idiotype IgM that binds with self-reactive NAAbs is postulated to neutralize pathogenicity [12]. Analysis of the relationship between NAAbs and autoimmune diseases might help in understanding the pathogenesis of autoimmune diseases.

Approaches for Detection and Analysis of NAAbs

Because a feline-specific immunoassay is barely available, hormonal research in cats is generally performed using assay systems developed for other species. However, many of them are inaccurate or completely useless. Previously, species differences were assumed to be the reason for this failure because of differences in amino acid composition of the analyte. Recently, we reported the presence of anti-insulin NAAbs in healthy cats [17]. Our results showed that NAAbs in healthy cats could be an important factor for the failure of immunoassay. In the reported study, we took advantage of several detection methods for NAAbs. We focused on the method of detection and analysis of NAAbs, which have been excluded as a background in the assay of pathogenic autoantibodies.

We tried to apply the assay kit originally developed for rat insulin (Shibayagi, Gunma, Japan) for determining feline serum insulin concentration. This kit employs sandwich ELISA, which contains anti-rat insulin antibodies for capturing and detecting antibodies. Initially, our attempt to determine feline serum insulin concentrations with the kit failed because every serum samples showed very low absorbance in ELISA. However, the assay system could determine the quantity of insulin purified from feline pancreas. Later, we found that the assay failed to measure insulin levels when feline serum was added to each well (Figure 1), thereby suggests the presence of inhibitory substances in feline serum.

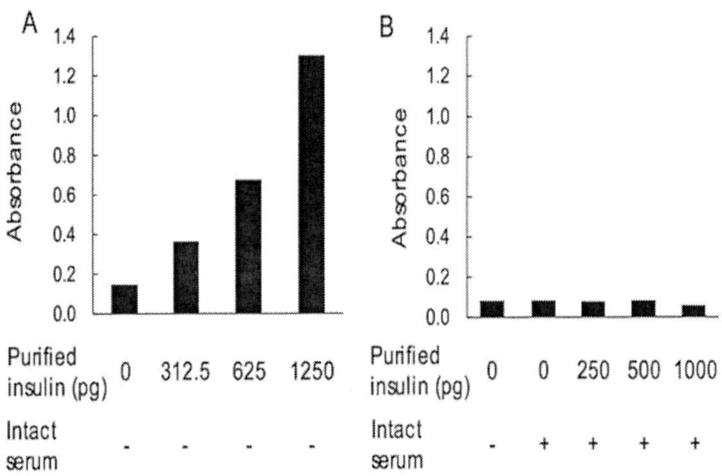

Figure 1. The interference with the ELISA system for insulin concentration..The ELISA for rat insulin was able to detect purified feline insulin, but failed in the presence of cats serum. Purified feline insulin concentration was determined by ELISA without (A) or with (B) addition of serum from healthy cats. Data are shown as mean (n=2) (From Nishii N et al. Domest Anim Endocrinol 38, 138-145, 2010.).

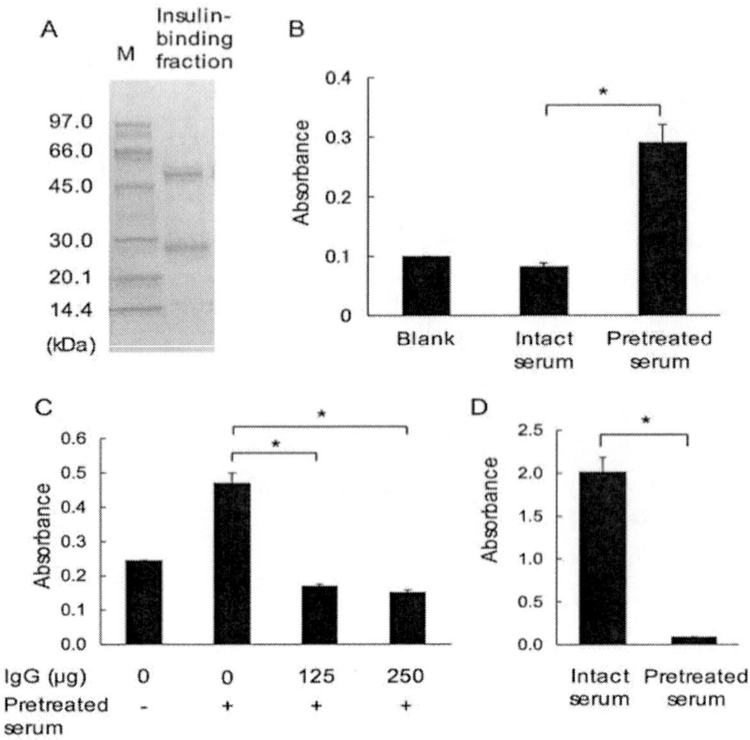

Figure 2. Involvement of insulin-binding IgG from healthy cats in interference with feline insulin assay. (A) SDS-PAGE for eluted insulin-bound fraction of affinity chromatography. (B) Pretreatment of serum samples for removing immunoglobulin increased the absorbance in the ELISA. Data are shown as means ± SEM. *P<0.05 (n=5). (C) An addition of purified insulin-binding IgG from healthy cats inhibited the insulin assay in pretreated serum samples. Data are shown as means ± SEM. *P<0.05 (n=4). (D) Insulin-IgG complex was measured in intact and pretreated serum. Data are shown as means ± SEM. *P<0.01 (n=10). (From Nishii N et al. Domest Anim Endocrinol 38, 138-145, 2010.)

Next, we proved that insulin-binding antibodies interfered in the assay for feline insulin concentrations. First, insulin-binding fraction of serum from healthy cats was obtained by affinity chromatography with bovine insulin. Bovine insulin (Sigma, St. Louis, MO, USA) was used because it has high amino-acid sequence homology with feline insulin and is commercially available. Bovine insulin was immobilized in coupling gel (CNBr-activated Sepharose 4B, GE Healthcare, Chalfont St. Giles, UK). Using bovine insulin-coupled sepharose gel, affinity chromatography was perfoemed. The serum sample was diluted with phosphate-buffered saline (PBS) up to a ratio of 1,1000, and then applied to the column. The column was subsequently washed with 10-fold column volumes of PBS. Insulin-bound molecules were then eluted with glycine-HCl. Insulin-bound fractions were collected and neutralized and then applied to SDS-PAGE (Figure 2A). SDS-PAGE showed clear biphasic bands 25 and 50 kDa in size, which was consistent with immunoglobulin.

From these results, we inferred that immunoglobulin removal enables the determination of feline serum insulin concentrations via ELISA. To remove immunoglobulin, serum samples were pretreated using a method that involved ammonium sulfate precipitation. This pretreatment effectively removed high molecular weight substances from feline serum samples, but barely affected serum insulin, which was confirmed by SDS-PAGE. In insulin ELISA, the absorbance of pretreated serum samples was significantly higher than that of intact serum (Figure 2B), which suggested that the pretreatment successfully removed the interfering substances from the serum. To confirm that the interfering substance was immunoglobulin, insulin-binding IgG was added to the pretreated serum samples followed by measurement of insulin concentrations (Figure 2C). The insulin-binding IgG was purified from the insulin-binding fraction using affinity chromatography with a protein A column (HiTrap Protein A HP column, GE healthcare). The addition of insulin-binding IgG significantly decreased absorbance in the assay. This evidence suggested that insulin-binding IgG interfered with ELISA for the measurement of feline serum insulin concentrations in healthy cats. NAAbs against insulin disturbed the immunoassay for insulin in cats. Feline NAAbs against insulin was present in a combined state with insulin, which was proved by sandwich ELISA (Figure 2D). In ELISA, anti-rat insulin antibody and horseradish peroxidase-labeled anti-feline IgG antibody were used for the capture and the detection of the insulin-IgG complex, respectively (Figure 3). The insulin-IgG complex correctly disappeared after pretreatment of the serum samples.

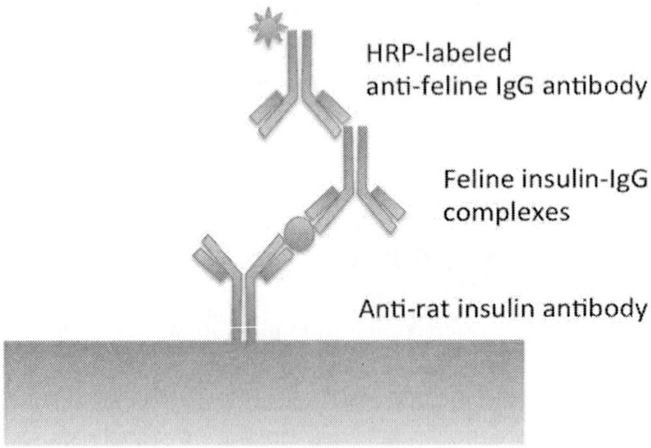

Figure 3. Scheme of the sandwich ELISA for the feline insulin-IgG complex. The plate was coated with anti-rat insulin antibodies, and the insulin-IgG complex was detected by HRP-labeled anti-feline IgG antibodies.

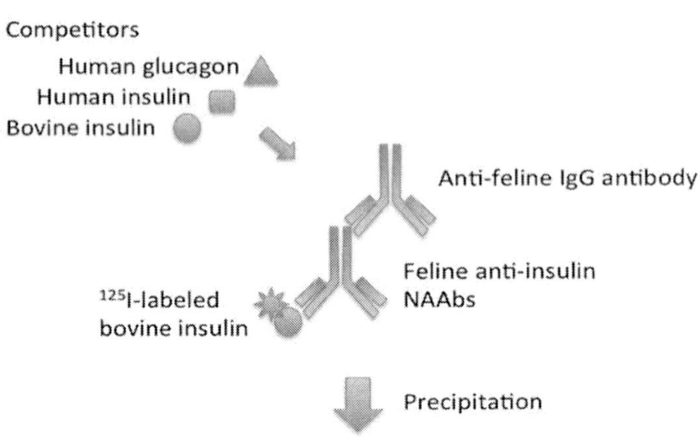

Figure 4. Scheme of radioimmunoassay for the analysis of the feline anti-insulin NAAbs. DCC-treated serum was incubated with 125I labeled bovine insulin. Bound 125I insulin was precipitated by adding anti-cat IgG antibody diluted with polyethyleneglycol solution, followed by centrifugation. Unlabeled bovine insulin, human insulin, and human glucagon were used as competitors.

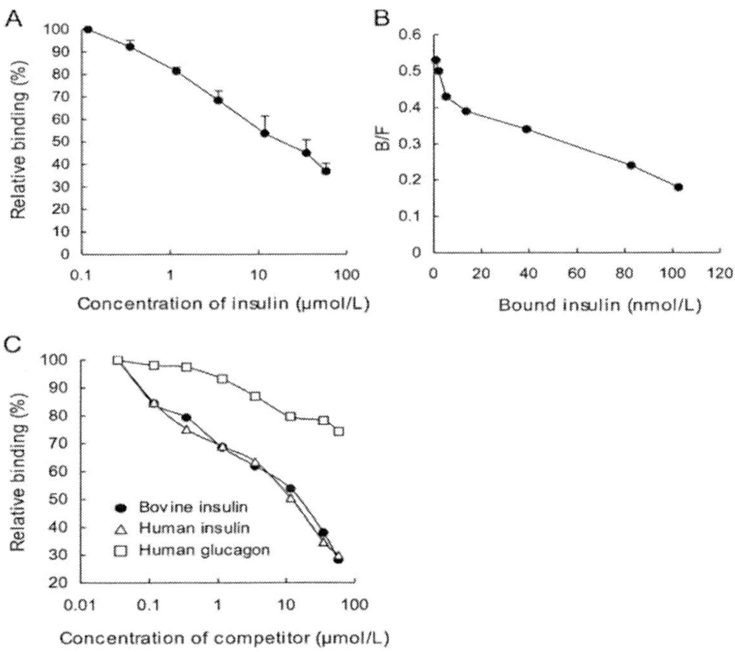

Figure 5. The competitive radioimmunoassay using 125I-bovine insulin for characterization of anti-insulin NAAbs in cats. (A) Displacement by unlabeled bovine insulin. Data are shown as means ± SEM of 6 samples with triplicate assay. (B) One of the samples that shows typical curvilinear nature in Scatchard plot analysis. (C) Specificity of the anti-insulin NAAbs in a cat. (From Nishii N et al. Domest Anim Endocrinol 38, 138-145, 2010.)

To analyze the characteristics of feline anti-insulin NAAbs, binding affinity and capacity was measured by competitive radioimmunoassay. For radioimmunoassay, bovine insulin was radiolabeled with 125I by the lactoperoxidase method [23]. Before the assay, serum samples were treated with acid dextran-coated charcoal (DCC) to remove low molecular substances [8]. This step excludes the effect of endogenous insulin, and enables the analysis of the properties of whole anti-insulin NAAbs. DCC solution was prepared from 0.25% w/v dextran and 2.5% w/v activated charcoal. One ml of serum was incubated for 25 min with 0.3 ml of 1N hydrochloric acid and 2.5 ml of DCC solution, and then neutralized with 0.2 ml of 0.5 N sodium hydrate solution. After centrifugation, the precipitation was removed. DCC-treated serum was incubated for 20 hours at 4°C with 125I labeled bovine insulin with or without unlabeled bovine insulin (Figure 4). PBS with 0.5% bovine serum albumin and 0.01% Triton X-100 was used as the reaction solution. Bound 125I insulin was precipitated by adding anti-cat IgG antibody diluted at 1,3000 with 3.5% polyethyleneglycol solution followed by centrifugation. This assay condition was decided based on preliminary experiments and may differ from antigen to antigen. Radioactivity was counted using a gammacounter. The binding of 125I labeled insulin was displaced with adding of unlabeled insulin (Figure 5A). Since Scatchard plot analysis showed a curvilinear pattern (Figure 5B), the data were analyzed by the 2-binding site model [18]. Calculation of association constants (Ka) and binding capacities (Bmax) suggested that anti-insulin NAAbs are relatively high in affinity and quantity. In addition, competition with human insulin and human glucagon showed that anti-insulin NAAbs have a certain level of specificity (Figure 5C). In these radioimmunoassays, the most important assignment was reducing background level, which was obtained by adjusting Triton X-100 concentration in the reaction buffer, coating assay plastic tubes, and precipitation method (eg. polyethyleneglycol concentration). Finally, Triton X-100 concentration was found to be the most important factor in reducing the background level.

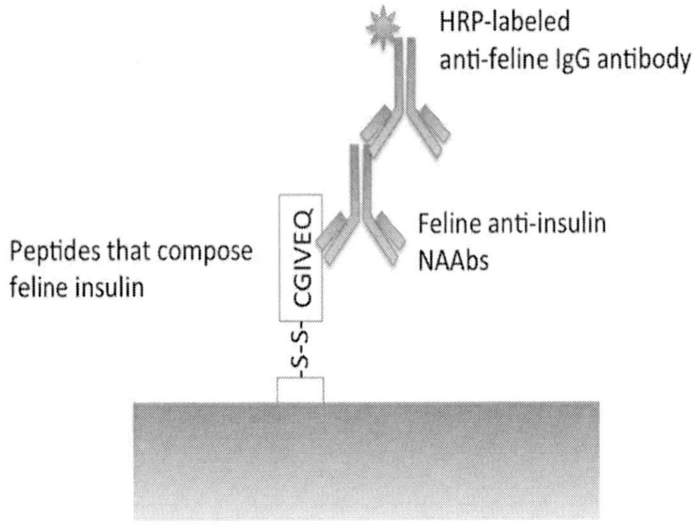

Figure 6. Scheme of the sandwich ELISA for the epitope analysis of feline anti-insulin NAAbs. The plate was coated with 12 synthesized peptides, and feline serum IgG was detected by HRP-labeled anti-feline IgG antibody.

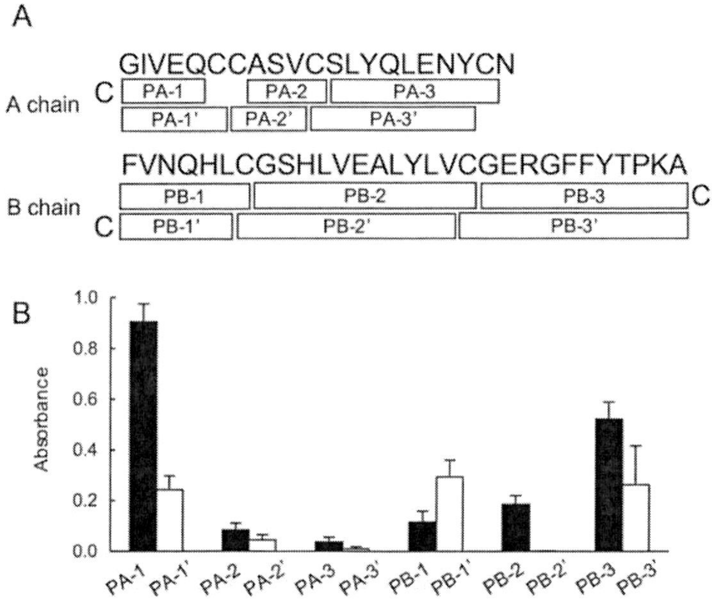

Figure 7. The epitope analysis of feline anti-insulin NAAbs. (A) Amino acid sequence of feline insulin molecule and 12 synthesized peptides consisting of feline insulin protein. (B) Binding of feline serum IgG to the synthesized peptides. Data are shown as means ± SEM (n=6). (From Nishii N et al. Domest Anim Endocrinol 38, 138-145, 2010.).

Next, we wanted to study the binding sites of anti-insulin NAAbs. To investigate the epitope, we employed ELISA, which consists of plates coated with a synthetic peptide composing feline insulin. Because the direction of peptides can affect the binding of NAAbs, the peptide was fused to the plate (Sulfhydryl Binding Plate, Corning, NY, USA) through sulfhydryl residue of cysteine (Figure 6). Each synthesized peptide contains cysteine at the end so that peptides can bind in a particular direction (Figure 7A). This artifice might not be essential, but it enabled analysis of the epitope. Bound anti-insulin NAAbs were detected with horseradish peroxidase-labeled anti-cat IgG antibody. Another ingenuity in this assay was the use of a commercial reaction solution (Can Get Signal, Toyobo, Osaka, Japan). This significantly improved sensitivity and specificity of the assay. The epitope analysis of anti-insulin NAAbs revealed that insulin residues A1-5 and B20-30 showed greater binding (Figure 7B). There were fewer individual differences in the binding pattern, which was consistent with the previous report [12].

Conclusion

NAAbs circulate in the blood of healthy individuals and may have various biological roles, including immunological defense, immunoregulation, and scavenging. Investigation of NAAbs possibly clarifies the enigma of immunology, such as immunological tolerance and pathology of autoimmune diseases. For the analysis of NAAbs, it is essential for researchers to establish a sensitive assay with low background activity.

References

[1] Avrameas, S. (1991). Natural autoantibodies, from 'horror autotoxicus' to 'gnothi seauton'. Immunol Today 12, 154-159.

[2] Avrameas, S. and Ternynck, T. (1995). Natural autoantibodies, the other side of the immune system. Res Immunol 146, 235-248.

[3] Baumgarth, N., Herman, O. C., Jager, G. C., Brown, L., Herzenberg, L. A. and Herzenberg, L. A. (1999). Innate and acquired humoral immunities to influenza virus are mediated by distinct arms of the immune system. Proc Natl Acad Sci USA 96, 2250-2255.

[4] Baumgarth, N., Tung, J. W. and Herzenberg, L. A. (2005). Inherent specificities in natural antibodies, a key to immune defense against pathogen invasion. Springer Semin Immun 26, 347-362.

[5] Casali, P., Burastero, S. E., Nakamura, M., Inghirami, G. and Notkins, A. L. (1987). Human lymphocytes making rheumatoid factor and antibody to ssDNA belong to Leu-1+ B-cell subset. Science 236, 77-81.

[6] Cui, Z., Zhao, M. H., Segelmark, M. and Hellmark, T. (2010). Natural autoantibodies to myeloperoxidase, proteinase 3, and the glomerular basement membrane are present in normal individuals. Kidney Int 78, 590-597.

[7] Galili, U., Clark, M. R. and Shohet, S. B. (1986). Excessive binding of natural anti-alpha-galactosyl immunoglobin G to sickle erythrocytes may contribute to extravascular cell destruction. *J. Clin. Invest.* 77, 27-33.

[8] Gerbitz, K. D. and Kemmler, W. (1978). Method for rapid quantitation and characterization of insulin antibodies. Clin Chem 24, 890-894.

[9] Hansen, M. B., Svenson, M., Abell, K., Yasukawa, K., Diamant, M. and Bendtzen, K. (1995). Influence of interleukin-6 (IL-6) autoantibodies on IL-6 binding to cellular receptors. Eur *J Immunol* 25, 348-354.

[10] Hayakawa, K., Asano, M., Shinton, S. A., Gui, M., Allman, D., Stewart, C. L., Silver, J. and Hardy, R. R. (1999). Positive selection of natural autoreactive B cells. Science 285, 113-116.

[11] Lacroix-Desmazes, S., Mouthon, L., Coutinho, A. and Kazatchkine, M. D. (1995). Analysis of the natural human IgG antibody repertoire, life-long stability of reactivities towards self antigens contrasts with age-dependent diversification of reactivities against bacterial antigens. Eur *J Immunol* 25, 2598-2604.

[12] Lacroix-Desmazes, S., Kaveri, S. V., Mouthon, L., Ayouba, A., Malanchère, E., Coutinho, A. and Kazatchkine, M. D. (1998). Self-reactive antibodies (natural autoantibodies) in healthy individuals. *J Immunol Methods* 216, 117-137.

[13] Lleo, A., Invernizzi, P., Gao, B., Podda, M. and Gershwin, M. E. (2010). Definition of human autoimmunity — autoantibodies versus autoimmune disease. Autoimmun Rev 9, A259-A266.

[14] Matsiota, P., Druet, P., Dosquet, P., Guilbert, B. and Avrameas, S. (1987). Natural autoantibodies in systemic lupus erythematosus. Clin Exp Immunol 69, 79-88.

[15] Mouthon, L., Nobrega, A., Nicolas, N., Kaveri, S. V., Barreau, C., Coutinho, A. and Kazatchkine, M. D. (1995). Invariance and restriction toward a limited set of self-antigens characterize neonatal IgM antibody repertoires and prevail in autoreactive repertoires of healthy adults. Proc Natl Acad Sci USA 92, 3839-3843.

[16] Naito, N., Saito, K., Hosoya, T., Tarutani, O., Sakata, S., Nishikawa, T., Niimi, H., Nakajima, H. and Kohno, Y. (1990). Anti-thyroglobulin autoantibodies in sera from patients with chronic thyroiditis and from healthy subjects, differences in cross-reactivity with thyroid peroxidase. Clin Exp Immunol 80, 4-10.

[17] Nishii, N., Takasu, M., Kojima, M., Hachisu, T., Wakabayashi, K., Iwasawa, A., Maeda, S., Ohba, Y. and Kitagawa, H. (2010). Presence of anti-insulin natural autoantibodies in healthy cats and its interference with immunoassay for serum insulin concentrations. Domest Anim Endocrinol 38, 138-145.

[18] Rosenthal, H. E. (1967). A graphic method for the determination and presentation of binding parameters in a complex system. Anal Biochem 20, 525-532.

[19] Rowley, B., Tang, L., Shinton, S., Hayakawa, K. and Hardy, R. R. (2007). Autoreactive B-1 B cells, constraints on natural autoantibody B cell antigen receptors. *J Autoimmun* 29, 236-245.

[20] Saadi, S. and Platt, J. L. (1995). Transient perturbation of endothelial integrity induced by natural antibodies and complement. *J Exp Med* 181, 21-

[21] Sabbaga, J., Pankewycz, O. G., Lufft, V., Schwartz, R. S. and Madaio, M. P. (1990). Cross-reactivity distinguishes serum and nephritogenic anti-DNA antibodies in human lupus from their natural counterparts in normal serum. *J Autoimmun* 3, 215-235.

[22] Sauerborn, M. and Schellekens, H. (2009). B-1 cells and naturally occurring antibodies, influencing the immunogenicity of recombinant human therapeutic proteins? Curr Opin Biotechnol 20, 715-721.

[23] Thorell, J. I. and Johansson, B. G. (1971). Enzymatic iodination of polypeptides with 125I to high specific activity. Biochim Biophys Acta 251, 363-369.

In: Autoantibodies
Editors: G. E. Jenkins and J. I. Hall

ISBN: 978-1-62081-560-1

Chapter VI

The Importance of Autoantibodies in the Etiology, Pathogenesis and Diagnosis of Autoimmune Diseases

Ali A. Al-Jabri*, Elias Said, Crystal Koh, Mohammed S. Al-Buloshi and Sidgi S. Hasson

Division of Immunology, Department of Microbiology and Immunology, College of Medicine and Health Sciences, Sultan Qaboos University, Muscat, Oman

Abstract

Antibodies that are directed against self antigens are called autoantibodies. Not all autoantibodies are harmful. Autoantibodies can be useful in the removal of cell debris during inflammation, and autoantibodies to inflammatory cytokines can protect against untoward inflammation. Some autoantibodies may be the actual pathogenetic agents of autoimmune disease, the secondary consequences of tissue damage, or the harmless footprints of an etiologic agent. They can also inform us about basic mechanisms of loss of tolerance and inflammation in patients with autoimmune diseases. Autoantibodies can be present

* Corresponding author: Professor Ali A. Al-Jabri, Head of Immunology Division Department of Microbiology and Immunology, College of Medicine and Health Sciences, Sultan Qaboos University, P. O. Box 35, Al Khod, Muscat Oman, Tel: 00968-24141186, Tel: 00968-24141186, Fax: 00968-24413419, E.mail: aaljabri@squ.edu.om

before the onset of some autoimmune diseases, show remarkable specificity and serve as biomarkers providing an opportunity for diagnosis and therapeutic intervention. Titers of some autoantibodies are increased in infections and in a variety of autoimmune diseases and are of little help in the differential diagnosis of disease. By contrast, most of the autoantibodies found in systemic autoimmune diseases are not detected in chronic infections. A negative result for antinuclear antibody (ANA) makes the diagnosis of systemic lupus or other systemic autoimmune disease unlikely, whereas a positive test with a high titer strongly supports the diagnosis. Likewise, in contrast to the high sensitivity and low specificity of rheumatoid factors (RFs) for rheumatoid arthritis, the anti-CCP autoantibody generally has a sensitivity of approximately 50%, but the specificity might be as high as 98%. Approximately 90% of patients with undifferentiated arthritis and raised anti-CCP auto-antibody titers will develop rheumatoid arthritis within few years. The specificity of many auto-antibodies has great diagnostic utility and might also have predictive value, such as with anti-CCP autoantibodies in rheumatoid arthritis. The specificity of autoantibodies in systemic auto-immunity also suggests an intimate relationship with disease pathogenesis. Few autoantibodies can be used alone to diagnose an autoimmune disease, because individuals without overt clinical disease, particularly relatives of patients with autoimmune diseases, might have detectable titers. Furthermore, some autoantibodies, although highly specific, are present only in a minority of patients. For example, autoantibodies to Smith occur in <30% of patients with systemic lupus. For these reasons, detection of autoantibodies is usually used to confirm a clinical diagnosis or help to define a subset of patients within a diagnostic category. In this chapter we discuss, the roles played by autoantibodies in the etiology, pathogenesis and diagnosis of autoimmune diseases with reference to our own experience in this field.

Keywords: Autoantibodies, Etiology, Autoimmune Disease, Diagnosis, Pathogenesis

1. INTRODUCTION

When the immune system's recognition apparatus breaks down, the body begins to produce antibodies and T cells directed against the body's own constituents-cells, cell components, or specific organs (Waldner 2009). These antibodies are known as autoantibodies. Autoantibodies react with self-antigens that may be found in all cell types (e.g. chromatin, centromeres) or be highly specific for a specific cell type in one organ of the body (e.g.

thyroglobulin in cells of the thyroid gland). They may comprise proteins, nucleic acids, carbohydrates, lipids or various combinations of these. Autoantibodies may be the actual pathogenetic agents of autoimmune disease, the secondary consequences of tissue damage, or the harmless footprints of an etiologic agent (Lleo et al. 2010)

Autoantibodies can be present in sera of patients with or without autoimmune diseases (Al-Jabri et al. 2003, Al-Jabri et al. 2004). The literature clearly defines their role in specific autoimmune conditions. Their presence merely supports, not confirms the diagnosis of an autoimmune disease; for a clinical diagnosis, evidence for clinical disease and/or tissue damage should be present. The definition of abnormality related to autoantibody levels is usually based on abnormal quantity rather than affinity or avidity. Thus, abnormal autoantibody levels can result in clinical or sub-clinical autoimmune conditions. The demonstration and interpretation of autoantibodies in sera from patients is a diagnostic tool in autoimmune diseases. Thus, the availability of data on the frequency and strength of autoantibodies within a normal population is important for determination of diagnostic levels (Al-Jabri et al. 2003). Theoretically, autoantibodies might be neutral or have beneficial or harmful effects. For example, while autoantibodies to thyroglobulin might not make a critical contribution to thyroiditis, long-acting thyroid stimulators (i.e. autoantibodies to the thyroid stimulating hormonr-TSH receptor) are responsible for thyrotoxicosis. Autoantibodies might be useful in the removal of cell debris during inflammation, and autoantibodies to inflammatory cytokines might protect against untoward inflammation (Elkon and Casali 2008).

2. The Physiological Roles of Autoantibodies in Healthy Individuals

Not all autoantibodies are harmful; some types appear to be integral to the immune system's regulatory scheme. Throughout life, our body continually generates autoantibodies (natural) which can recognize self and non-self as well as foreign antigens. These natural autoantibodies are produced at tightly regulated levels in the complete absence of external antigenic stimulation. They are produced mainly, if not exclusively, by a subset of long-lived, self-replenishing B cells, known as B-1 cells or $CD5^+$ B cells (Sauerborn and Schellekens 2009). Autoantibodies remained ignored until the appearance of the immune network theory which postulates that the immune system of healthy individuals can produce antibodies to a variety of antigens of their own body (Lacroix-Desmazes et al. 1998). Experimental supports to this theory confirms the presence of such autoantibodies in the blood serum of healthy persons, specifically directed to hormones, receptors, intercellular matrix components, cytoskeletal proteins, DNA, histones, enzymes, components of the main histocompatibility complex, and other endogenic compounds.

It has been proposed that autoantibodies function primarily to control autoreactivity and immune homeostasis, in healthy individuals (Sauerborn and Schellekens 2009). These antibodies seem to have an important role in the innate immune system, as first line of defense against pathogens as well as in the prevention of autoimmune diseases ((Waldner 2009, Sauerborn and Schellekens 2009). In addition, autoantibodies have a high affinity to carbon groups present in the membrane of many microbes and by binding to pathogens, antigen–antibody complexes can induce complement mediated lysis. They also have a crucial influence on protecting the body against waste products and clear the body from apoptotic process (Lacroix-Desmazes et al. 1998, Sauerborn and Schellekens 2009). Recently, several functions have been attributed to natural autoantibodies, clearance of aging cells, anti-tumoral surveillance, anti-inflammatory activity, selection of immune repertoires and homeostasis of autoreactivity (Sauerborn and Schellekens 2009).

3. The Role of Autoantibodies in the Etiology of Autoimmune Diseases

The presence of autoantibodies is not necessary associated with a disease (Al-Jabri et al. 2003, Al-Jabri et al. 2004); however autoantibodies can be dangerous when they attack body tissues causing their damage, hence being an important part of autoimmune disease players. Autoantibodies are implicated in the majority of autoimmune diseases and sometimes they play the major role in the pathogenesis.

3.1. Development of B-Lymphocytes

B-lymphocytes producing autoantibodies are supposed to be deleted, during the development of these cells in a process called the central tolerance, or after they become mature B-cells in a process called peripheral tolerance. However, some of these cells can escape these processes and participate in autoimmune diseases.

Immature B-lymphocytes develop in the bone marrow from hematopoietic stem cells. Stem cells differentiate to Pro-B cells expressing CD19 and CD10. The D_H gene segment is rearranged to J_H gene segment in these cells. The pro-B cell differentiates to Pre-B cell who also express CD19 and CD10 and have a VDJ unit formed after the rearrangement of the V_H gene segment. A pre-B cell express on its surface the μ chain, linked to the VpreB and λ5 genes products. The μ chain is adjacent to Igα (CD79a) and Igβ (CD79b) molecules forming together the pre-B-cell-receptor. When the B-cell reaches the immature stage it expresses a monomeric IgM on its surface together with Igα and Ig$\beta\alpha$ and it becomesCD20$^+$. In this stage if the B-cell is able to recognize self-antigens expressed on the surface of cells from the bone marrow, it undergoes receptor editing to change its light chain and thus change its specificity in order to prevent the generation of antibodies that interact with self-antigens. When the new specificity is still targeting a self-antigen, the B-cell dies by apoptosis and thus it is deleted in a process called the negative selection. The survived immature B-cells will differentiate to mature B-cells expressing both IgM and IgD on their surface. This process of development allows the generation of B-cells with a broad spectrum of specificity. At this stage, when B-cells interact with antigens they will be activated and will produce antibodies having a single specificity and a single isotype. These cells are called plasma cells and they do not express Ig molecules or the above mentioned CD molecules on their surface. An activated mature B-cell can also differentiate to a memory B-cell, expressing IgG, IgE or IgA and CD27 on their surface, this cell will not proliferate but it will respond to further activations (Schelonka et al. 2010, Nescakova et al. 2011).

3.2. B-Cell Tolerance

To avoid damages caused by autoantibodies produced by self-reacting B-cells, the latter should be self-tolerant hence they should not be activated in response to self-antigens. The self-tolerance is achieved by two phenomenon; the central tolerance occurring in the early stages of B-cells development in the bone marrow, and the peripheral tolerance which occurs after a mature B-cell leaves the bone marrow. The aim of the central tolerance is to allow the survival of B-cells specific for foreign antigens only. However, when autoreactive B-cells escape they are controlled by the peripheral tolerance to avoid the production of autoantibodies. The central tolerance has several mechanisms such as: receptor editing and deletion as mentioned above; anergy, where the B-cell is inactivated and will not respond to further activation; clonal ignorance, where auto reactive B-cell can escape other tolerance mechanisms because the antigen is present in low concentrations or because of the low affinity of the BCR, thus these cells will not be stimulated to produce autoantibodies (Sandel et al. 1999, Yarkoni et al. 2010).

Some autoreactive B-cells are able to escape these mechanisms or to change specificity in the periphery to recognize self-antigens, hence they should be controlled by mechanisms of the peripheral tolerance such as: anergy due to the lack of a second signal provided by T-cells when a B-cell recognize a self-antigen, e.g. the signal provided by CD40 ligand expressed on T helper cells through CD40 expressed on B-cells; ignorance where autoreactive B-cells are capable of making a response but are unaware of the presence of their auto-antigen because of its low concentration or because of its presence in locations which are not freely exposed to surveillance; T-regulatory cells, which can suppress B-cell function (Monson 2008, Yarkoni et al. 2010). Some autoreactive B-cells can still escape these mechanisms and they can produce autoantibodies causing autoimmune diseases. This is caused by genetic and environmental factors.

3.3. Factors Regulating Autoantibodies Production

There is a familial tendency for autoimmune diseases and the incidence increase in the monozygotic twins (Barcellos et al. 2006). Despite some cases where a single gene can be responsible for the autoimmune diseases, the latter are commonly caused by a combination of several genes. The abnormal expression of some genes is associated with autoimmune diseases and autoantibodies production, these genes are implicated in apoptosis and survival, such as Fas, FasL, BAFF, and BCL-2; BCR signaling, such as CD22, lyn, SHP-1 and CD19 (Dörner et al. 2006); cytokine expression such as IL-17, TNF-α and IFN-α, and costimulation, such as CD40 and CD40L (Tincani et al. 2007; Felix et al. 2010, Mountz et al. 2011). Although the antibody repertoire appear randomly divers, the use of gen segments is nonrandom. Tendencies to use some gene segments in a population can be related to autoimmune diseases, as they will result in an abnormal development of B-cells (Kipps et al. 1989, Damle et al. 2000).

The abnormalities in gene sequences coding for antibodies can result in autoantibodies that are abnormal in their specificity and composition, such as anti-double-stranded DNA antibodies that have mutations in the HCDR3 region (Shlomchik et al. 1990).

While receptor editing is supposed to prevent the production of irregular antibodies, it can introduce abnormalities leading to the production of autoantibodies (Meffre et al. 2000, Hansen et al. 2000).Some factors can be dependent on the rate of availability of antigens in the different organs and on the capacity to eliminate apoptosis products in the body (Holdenrieder et al. 2006).

Other factors that can initiate autoimmune diseases depend on environmental infectious or noninfectious factors. These factors can lead to the exposure of some self-antigens that were hidden in immune-privileged sites and to which autoreactive B-cells exist (Liao et al. 1995, Malmstrom et al. 1997, Malmstrom et al. 1998). Some antibodies directed against foreign antigens, able of inducing an immune response, can cross-interact with self-antigens, which originally were not able to trigger an immune response, because of the presence of similar epitopes in both antigens, this phenomenon is called molecular mimicry (Bogdanos et al. 2001, Wucherpfennig et al. 2001, Racanelli et al. 2011). Idiotype cross-reaction can also influence the production of autoantibodies. Indeed, autoimmunity can be induced because of cross-reaction between an anti-idiotype of an antibody, directed against a virus, and the receptor of this virus on the cells of the host (Tzioufas et al. 2010).

The polyclonal activation of B-cells with pathogen-associated molecular patterns (PAMPS) can lead to the induction of autoimmune antibodies production by B-cells. For instance, B-cells can be activated by LPS via TLR4, by CpG DNA via TLR9 or by signle stranded RNA (ssRNA) via TLR7 and TLR8 (Green et al. 2011). Polyclonal activation of B-cells can also occur through super-antigens upon infection with some organisms (Wucherpfennig et al. 2001).

The production of autoantibodies can be activated by hormones and it can be gender-dependent in some cases such as the influence of estrogen in SLE (Cutolo et al. 2009, Cunningham et al. 2011). Some drugs can modify the self-antigen and render them more immunogenic such as penicillin, α-methyldopa, hydralazine and procainamide (Whittingham et al. 1976, Kirtland HH 3rd et al. 1980, Smiley et al. 1988).

4. The Role of Autoantibodies in the Pathogenesis of Autoimmune Diseases

The disease-causing injury can be mediated by autoantibodies and/or by autoreactive T cells in autoimmune disorders, and the extent of autoantibody-mediated pathogenesis varies depending on the autoimmune disease. For instance, autoantibodies play the essential role in pathogenesis in autoimmune hemolytic anemia and systemic lupus erythematosus (SLE) whereas autoreactive T cell-mediated destruction of insulin-producing β cells of the pancreatic islets is the central mechanism of pathogenesis in type 1 diabetes (T1D). While one arm of the adaptive immune responses may play a major role in different autoimmune diseases, the roles of humoral and cell-mediated immunity are not mutually exclusive since T cell help is essential for production of pathogenic autoantibodies and antigen presentation by B cells to autoreactive $CD4^+$ T cells is necessary for optimal T cell activation. The presence of autoantibodies does not always lead to development of autoimmune diseases as autoantibodies are present in healthy individuals (Al-Shukaili and Al-Jabri 2006). Autoantibodies of IgM isotype are secreted by short-lived plasma cells that have differentiated from naïve B cells responding to the autoantigens and have low affinity to the autoantigens. On the other hand, IgG autoantibodies are produced by activated and/or memory B cells or long-lived plasma cells, which have undergone isotype-switching and affinity maturation (Walport 2001a, Walport 2001b, Yanaba et al. 2008). Majority of the autoantibodies with a greater pathogenic capacity in autoimmunity is IgG isotype.

A wide array of autoantibodies against various self antigens may be formed in autoimmunity, but not all autoantibodies are involved in inducing tissue injury. However, when pathogenic autoantibodies bind to self antigens, they can induce activation of the complement cascade and FcγR-expressing mononuclear phagocytes leading to a direct lysis or depletion of cells bearing the antigen or can elicit inflammatory responses causing the tissue destruction (Walport 2001a, Walport 2001b, Nimmerjahn and Ravetch 2006). Activation of the complement and phagocytic systems as well as induction of inflammatory responses are the protective mechanisms against invading pathogens. However, persistent immune responses to autoantigens, which cannot be eliminated and thus amplify the responses, lead to high levels of autoantibodies and isotype switching of autoantibodies to IgG isotypes. These autoantibodies binding to cell surface or extracellular matrix antigens ultimately induce type II hypersensitivity reactions causing destruction or dysfunction of cells and tissues. Additionally, autoantibodies against soluble self antigens form immune complexes, which induce type III hypersensitity reactions with chronic inflammation causing tissue damages. In the sections to follow, specific mechanisms of autoantibody-mediated pathogenesis and their examples are discussed.

4.1. Autoantibody-Mediated Cellular Destruction

Autoantibodies can develop against cell-surface or extracellular matrix antigens and elicit type II hypersensitivity reactions that cause cellular destruction. Autoantibodies of IgM and IgG isotypes binding to cell surface antigens activate the complement system, and this can lead to formation of the membrane attack complex (MAC) causing direct lysis of the target cells. Alternatively, complement protein subunits, such as C3b, that are generated during the complement activation process and bind to the target cell surface, render them to be cleared by complement receptor-mediated phagocytosis (Walport 2001a, Walport 2001b). IgG autoantibody-sensitized cells can also be destroyed by FcγR-mediated mechanisms; phagoctyes and natural killer (NK) cells express FcγRs, and the target cells are rapidly cleared by FcγR-mediated phagocytosis or antibody-dependent cell-mediated cytotoxicity (ADCC) respectively (Rodien et al. 1996; Frisoni et al. 2005;). Type II hypersensitivity reactions are frequently observed in various autoimmune diseases, and hemolytic anemia is an example. IgG or IgM antibodies bind to autoantigens on red blood cells leading to either a direct lysis by the complement system or by depletion from the blood via the mononuclear phagocytic system resulting in anemia in the affected individuals (Silberstein 1993, Clynes and Ravetch 1995, Domen 1998).

While red blood cells are effectively lysed by the complement system, mammalian nucleated cells are usually resistant to complement-mediated lysis due to soluble and cell membrane-bound proteins, which regulate activities of various complement components (Schieren and Hansch 1993, Meri and Jarva 1998). Therefore, complement-mediated lysis of nucleated cells such as neutrophils, platelets, and lymphocytes are relatively rare; however, when these cells are coated with autoantibodies, depletion can still occur via phagocytosis and ADCC. For example, autoantibodies against GpIIb:IIIa fibrinogen receptor on platelets or other platelet-specific surface antigens can cause thrombocytopenia leading to hemorrhage in autoimmune thrombocytopenic purpura (Beardsley and Ertem 1998). The intravenous immunoglobulin (IVIG) treatment, which is the administration of non-specific IgG, is used as a part of therapy for certain autoimmunity, and the efficacy of IVIG treatment highlights the role of FcγR-mediated clearance of the autoantibody-coated cells (Shoenfeld and Katz 2005). Regardless of the mechanisms of cellular destruction, resulting pathology is due to the depletion of cells via rapid clearance from the body.

4.2. Autoantibody-Induced Inflammation and Tissue Damage

Autoantibodies to tissue or extracellular matrix antigens can stimulate local inflammatory responses, which can be amplified via various mechanisms causing tissue damage. When the complement system is activated by IgG and IgM autoantibodies bound to tissue antigens, a number of soluble subunits of the complement components is generated including C3a and C5a. They are powerful chemoattractants recruiting inflammatory cells, including neutrophils, macrophages, basophils, and mast cells, to the tissue (Nakagawa and Komorita 1993). C3a and C5a can also activate endothelial cells and mast cells in the tissue to produce other chemotactic factors. Once recruited to the tissue, the inflammatory leukocytes are further activated by the cell membrane-bound subunits of the complement components or Fc portion of the autoantibodies bound to tissue antigens via complement or Fcγ receptors, respectively. Activated leukocytes can then release a variety of cytokines and toxic lipid mediators, and these products of inflammatory responses as well as ADCC cause the tissue injury.

One example of this type of autoimmunity is Goodpasture's syndrome, in which autoantibodies against basement membrane collagen (type IV collagen) bind to the glomerular basement membranes or to the basement membranes of pulmonary alveoli and induce inflammation in the kidney or lungs, respectively.

The local inflammation rapidly recruits inflammatory leukocytes to the target tissue, and activation of monocytes, neutrophils, and tissue mast cells by FcγR cross-linking by the autoantibodies bound to basement membrane amplify further recruitment of these cells and release of large amount of inflammatory cytokines and lipid mediators causing severe damage to the kidney or lungs that can be fatal if untreated (Ooi et al. 2008).

Another example of autoimmune diseases, in which pathology is due to autoantibody-induced inflammation, is pemphigus vulagaris. Patients with pemphigus vulgaris develop ulceration of the oral mucosa and extensive epidermal blisters because of inflammation-mediated injuries elicited by autoantibodies formed against desmosomes, which are responsible for adhesion between the cells in the epidermis (Amagai 2003).

4.3. Induction of Cellular Dysfunction by Autoantibodies to Receptors

The type II hypersensitivity reaction that is unique to autoimmunity and does not occur as a conventional defense mechanism against pathogens is induction of cellular dysfunction by autoantibodies against specific receptors expressed on cell surface.

The outcome of autoantibody-binding of a cell surface receptor is either inhibition or stimulation of the cellular function. Myasthenia gravis and Graves' disease are the classical examples of autoimmune diseases induced by inhibition or stimulation of a cell function respectively. In myasthenia gravis, neuromuscular transmission mediated by acetylcholine receptor expressed on skeletal muscle cells at neuromuscular junctions is impaired due to autoantibodies binding to the alpha chain of the receptor. Autoantibodies not only block the binding of the natural ligand, acetylcholine, but also triggers internalization of the receptor followed by intracellular degradation. Patients with myasthenia gravis develop muscle weakness, which can progress to a more severe form potentially fatal if untreated (Vincent et al. 1999, Meriggioli and Sanders 2009).

In contrast to myasthenia gravis, pathogenesis of Graves' disease involves autoantibodies against the thyroid-stimulating hormone (TSH) receptor on thyroid cells that stimulate the overproduction of thyroid hormone. Under the normal condition, thyroid hormones regulate TSH production by the pituitary via a negative-feedback mechanism: TSH stimulates thyroid cells via TSH receptor signaling to produce thyroid hormones, and consequent high levels of thyroid hormones shut down

TSH production, which in turn suppresses secretion of thyroid hormones. In Graves' disease, this negative-feedback loop fails, and thyroid cells continue to produce high levels of thyroid hormones because of continual stimulation of TSH receptors by the autoantibodies (Bahn and Heufelder 1993).

4.4. Systemic Tissue Destruction by Immune Complex-Mediated Inflammatory Responses

When antibodies are formed against soluble autoantigens, tissue injury can be caused by the autoantibody-soluble antigen immune complexes. Formation of immune complexes is a part of normal humoral immune responses, and when they are formed, they can bind complement components, which allow efficient clearance of the immune complexes by red blood cells via complement receptors and by mononuclear phagocytes via both complement and Fcγ receptors. Dead cells and apoptotic bodies are also removed by phagocytes, and this clearance occurs in the spleen and liver (Ravichandran and Lorenz 2007). However, when high levels of autoantibodies directed against soluble antigens are produced due to autoimmunity, these autoantibodies form immune complexes in large amount that can overwhelm the clearance system. In addition, failure to clear immune complexes as well as apoptotic cells due to a defect in the clearance mechanism is one of the major factors attributable to the onset and severity of immune complex-mediated autoimmune diseases (Gaipl et al. 2007, Lleo et al. 2008). Immune complexes, which are not cleared from the circulation, are deposited in various tissues and induce inflammation causing the tissue damage.

A classical example of immune complex-mediated autoimmune disease is SLE (Tan 1989, Kotzin 1996). In SLE, autoantibodies against wide range of soluble antigens, including endogenous nucleic acids and associated proteins, form immune complexes. Patients with SLE generally have high levels of anti-nuclear antigen and/or anti-double stranded DNA (dsDNA) antibodies as well as antibodies to various components of extractable nuclear antigens (ENA). Normally, these intracellular antigens are inaccessible to the antigen receptors and antibodies, but in SLE, they become detectable on dying cells and released from dead cells and damaged tissues. The continued extracellular availability of the autoantigens leads to continued stimulation of autoantibody production resulting in persistent formation of small immune complexes that are not efficiently cleared from the circulation. These immune complexes are deposited in various tissues including glomerular basement membrane of the kidney, joints, and/or endothelium of small blood vessels and activate inflammatory responses leading to influx of neutrophils and monocytes, which are further activated via Fcγ receptors. More autoantigens are released from the injured tissues into the extracellular milieu and amplify the autoantibody responses, immune complex formation, and inflammation (Singh 2005).

Ultimately, continued inflammation induced in the target tissues causes sufficient damage that can lead to significant morbidity and mortality.

4.5. Role of Autoantibodies in Cell-Mediated Autoimmune Diseases

Although certain autoimmune disease such as rheumatoid arthritis (RA), type 1 diabetes (T1D), and multiple sclerosis (MS) are generally considered to involve T cell-mediated pathology, recent studies suggest important roles of B cells and autoantibodies (Yanaba et al. 2008). RA is a chronic autoimmune disorder in which synovium of the joints is the main target of autoimmune-mediated inflammation and damage that are driven by T cells and macrophages. Rheumatoid factor (RF), autoantibody against Fc portion of human IgG, is found 70-80% of RA patients but is not specific to RA as it is also found in patients with other autoimmune diseases and in infections. Moreover, RF is present in up to 10% of healthy individuals (Sutton et al. 2000). However, there are qualitative differences between RF found in healthy individuals and RA patients. RF in healthy individuals is IgM-natural antibodies produced by B-1 B cells with low affinity and polyreactivity. In contrast, RF found in RA patients has undergone isotype switching, somatic hypermutation, and affinity maturation (Firestein 2003). Thus, pathogenic RF forms immune-complexes with IgG in the synovium and elicit inflammatory responses via FcγR-triggering and complement activation and recruits T cells and macrophages for amplification of the inflammation resulting in synovial tissue damage and progression of the disease. Autoantibodies to citrullinated proteins in the synovium environment have emerged as autoantibodies highly specific for RA; two-thirds of RA patients have autoantibodies against citrulline-modified proteins (anti-CCP) while they are very rare in healthy individuals (<2%) (Rantapaa-Dahlqvist et al. 2003, van Gaalen et al. 2005). However, the relevant targets of anti-CCP antibodies in joints and other peripheral tissues are currently unidentified, and their role in RA pathogenesis remains unclear.

Autoantibodies against various self antigens are also present in other T cell-mediated autoimmune diseases including T1D and MS. In pre-diabetic individuals as well as animal models of T1D, autoantibodies specific for β cells antigens are frequently detected before the onset of the disease and can predict development of the disease in susceptible individuals (Yu and Eisenbarth 2004). Similarly, presence of autoantibodies to myelin basic protein, myelin oligodendrocyte glycoprotein, and other central nervous system antigens have been observed in some MS patients (Cross et al. 2001). Studies using various animal models of T1D and MS [e.g. non-obese diabetic mouse models for T1D, experimental allergic encephalomyelitis in rat models] have indicated potential effects of the autoantibodies on pathology (Cross et al. 2001, Silveira and Grey 2006); nevertheless, it is unclear whether the autoantibodies actually participate in pathogenesis or their presence is simply an associating feature of the diseases in human.

5. The Roles of Autoantibodies in the Diagnosis of Autoimmune Diseases

Currently, autoimmunity laboratories are in a very dynamic situation owing to the constant and increasing availability of new and developed tests, mainly due to the detection of new autoantibodies and demonstration of their clinical usefulness. Continuous improvement of the biochemical and molecular methods has allowed rapid dissection of the autoantigens associated with specific autoimmune diseases.

The rheumatic and autoimmune diseases can generally be classified into two groups: those that are systemic in nature with varieties of autoantibodies which are highly specific for certain diseases, including anti-dsDNA, anti-Sm, anti-ribosomal P autoantibodies in SLE, anti-topoisomerase I (Scl-70) in scleroderma, anti-CCP in rheumatoid arthritis, anti-SS-A/Ro, anti-SS-B/La in Sjögren‘s syndrome (SjS), anti-U1-RNP, anti-PM-Scl in mixed connective tissue disease (MCTD) or anti-Jo-1 in polymyositis or dermatomyositis. And those that are more organ or tissue directed which are associated with autoantibodies specific to the main affected organ, like thyroglobulin (TGA) and thyroid peroxidase enzyme (TPO) in thyroiditis, insulin and glutamic acid decarboxilase autoantibodies in T1D and anti-mitochondrial autoantibody in primary billiary cirrhosis.

The detection of such autoantibodies may represent a status of disease activity or at least predict a future pathogenic condition. However, each of these groups presents unique problems to the diagnostic laboratory, complicated by the fact that they may occur in combination with each other. And this in return will reflect that the autoimmunity laboratories should analyze and measure an increasing number of autoantibodies employing a broad spectrum of techniques and methods (González-Buitrago and González

2006). On the other hand it has been clearly shown that autoantibodies that are associated with autoimmune diseases not only play a significant role as diagnostic markers, but that their occurrence may also be used to make a well-founded prediction. For example, in the past, when autoantibodies were found to be in a patient who apparently showed no signs of disease, this was generally assumed to be a false positive result at that time. However, thanks to some excellent studies done at that time which has been stored for documentation purposes, it is well known now that autoantibodies can occur 10 to 20 years before the outbreak of autoimmune disease, and in some cases even earlier. The most striking example of this is with primary biliary cirrhosis, where the typical anti-mitochondrial antibodies (AMA) may be identified 30 years before the occurrence of the first symptoms. Anti-dsDNA antibodies precede the development of SLE by 5 to 10 years.

5.1. The Role of the Autoimmunity Laboratory in Autoimmune Diseases

Autoimmunity laboratories use immunoassays as the basic technique for the determination of autoantibodies and not the antigens (González-Buitrago and González 2006). Important antigens have been well described and they are applied in methods that are used to detect autoantibodies. The detection from autoantibodies to antigens for examples; SS-A/Ro, SS-B/La, Sm, RNP, Scl-70, PM-Scl and Jo-1 are clinically useful in systemic autoimmune diseases. There are a number of other antigens which have been used in assays for the detection of autoantibodies associated with specific systemic or organ specific diseases. The clinical usefulness of the analysis' results depends on the quality of the laboratory tests. Hence an ideal diagnostics test has both, high sensitivity and specificity. It also identifies all patients with diseases and is not positive in those who do not have diseases (Bossuyt et al. 2004, Von PAJM et al. 2006).

5.2. Techniques Used for the Detection of Autoantibodies

Requests of screening tests for autoantibody detection have risen remarkably, mainly due to the increased understanding of the nature of autoantibodies. The main analytical techniques used in the autoimmunity laboratory are listed in Table 1.

Table 1. Analytical techniques used in the autoimmunity laboratory

Indurect Immunofluorescence (IIF)
Immunoassays
Enzyme immunoassays (ELISA)
IRMA
Immunoblot
Western blot
Dot blot
Agglutination (Haemagglutination and latex agglutination)
Immunoprecipitation
Turbidimetry
Nephelometry
Double immunodiffusion
Counterimmunoelectrophoresis

Over the last few years, the most significant trend at the autoimmunity laboratory has been the gradual replacement of microscopy (indirect immunofluorescence, IIF) and other manual methods such as double immunodiffusion and counter immuno-electrophoresis, by immunoassays such as enzyme immunoassay (EIA), which requires less skilled operators. This immunoassay is more objective, and can easily be automated. The following sections illustrate the common techniques that are in use nowadays in the autoimmunity laboratories.

5.3. Enzyme Immunoassay

At present, enzyme immunoassays offer a basic technique and it is widely used for identifying specific autoantibodies to nuclear or cytoplasmic antigens of different group of organ-specific disorders, such as Grave′s disease, primary biliary cirrhosis, insulin-dependent diabetes mellitus or systemic affecting different organs like systemic sclerosis, Sjögren's syndrome, mixed connective tissue disease or rheumatoid arthritis, in clinical laboratories (Jaskowski et al. 1996, Stinton and Fritzler 2007). Of the several different forms of enzyme immunoassays, the enzyme-linked immunosorbent assay (ELISA) format is the one most used.

ELISAs for \ANAs show good sensitivity and a high negative predictive value, so they can be used to eliminate samples without ANA, although because of their low positive predictive value, positive samples must be analysed by Indirect Immuno-Fluoresce to confirm the presence of ANA and to determine the final result.

However, it should be noted that new horizons are continually being found for EIA in the autoimmunity laboratory, addressing a question of whether this new era of ANA screening might mean farewell to the microscope Nossent and Rekvig 2001).

ELISA is also used to measure anti-dsDNA antibodies (Tan et al. 1999, Gonza'lez et al. 2004, Burlingame 2004). In general, anti-dsDNA ELISAs have very good diagnostic sensitivity, but with low diagnostic specificity, because they detect high- and low-avidity antibodies; the latter considered of low clinical relevance.

When using ELISA as a screening method for SLE for example, another test such as IIF should be used to increase diagnostic specificity, and/or the Farr assay, which only detect high-avidity antibodies. Nucleosomes have been considered a major autoantigen in SLE and the measurement of anti-nucleosome antibodies has been proposed as more sensitive and specific than that of antidsDNA antibodies for SLE and drug-induced lupus (Burlingame 2004, Gonza'lez-Buitrago et al. 2003).

Antinucleosome autoantibodies react with epitopes comprised of the native DNA structure found in chromatin, the native histone epitopes exposed in chromatin, and epitopes made up of the histone–DNA complex found in chromatin. Specifically excluded are reactivities to non-histone proteins such as centromere and DNA topoisomerase I (González-Buitrago et al. 2003). However, based on experience anti-nucleosome antibodies and antidsDNA antibodies provide similar information in established SLE (Sun et al. 1998). Currently ELISA is also being used for the measurement of anticentromere antibodies using recombinant antigen (Hoffman et al., 2002). Several ELISA methods have been described for the detection of anti-neutrophil cytoplasm antibodies, using purified and recombinant antigens. Attempts to obtain recombinant PR3 have not been successful for obtaining a protein reactive to human antibodies. Immobilisation of native PR3 by coating plastic plates can provide partial denaturation, with changes to conformational epitopes, which can produce a loss of reactivity with autoantibodies. This phenomenon has been observed in some patients treated with anti-PR3 antibodies and could be overcomed by using a capture monoclonal antibody to immobilize PR3 protein (Stinton and Fritzler 2007).

5.4. Immunofluorescence

The IIF technique, which uses various tissue sections or the human larynx epithelioma cell line (HEp-2) that have larger nuclei and nucleoli than rodent tissue cells as an antigenic source, has had major implications for the diagnosis of autoimmune diseases in a routine laboratory setting (Stinton and Fritzler 2007). Autoantibodies give characteristic fluorescence images called fluorescence patterns. The staining pattern provides some indication of the specificity of the antibodies in the sample. Hence the IIF staining pattern of a positive sample can be used to evaluate which appropriate antigen specificities to look for. In the first applications of this technique, slices with fixed tissues for example Hep-2 or from mouse or rat tissue were incubated with serum samples and the binding of serum autoantibodies to their corresponding antigens in the tissues is detected by using fluorescent-labelled anti-immunoglobulin antiserum. It is well known that the HEp-2 cells used for the detection of autoantibodies do not have a satisfactory ability to give positive IIF results for antibodies to SS-A/Ro-52 and Jo-1 (histidil-tRNA synthetase) (Hayashi et al 2001). Many serum samples give speckled or grainy homogenous staining patterns which cannot be clearly identified as one of the known patterns (Stinton and Fritzler 2007). Other drawbacks associated with IIF are the substrate variations, manual performance, subjective result interpretation, low reproducibility and a lack of standardisation. In order to overcome these limitations, there were some solutions being introduced. The first one is that for most IIF assays, the laboratory should select a screening dilution, because undiluted serum gives a background staining due to the non-specific binding of clinically non-significant levels of circulating autoantibodies. Increasing the screening dilution produces a less sensitive and more specific assay. However, the greater sensitivity of ANA assays with HEp-2 cells as compared to rodent tissues is associated with lower specificity. Thus, more patients with diseases other than SLE and healthy people show positive results. To overcome this problem a 1/160 titer has been recommended as the most acceptable cut off to separate normal from abnormal sera (Tan et al. 1997).

IIF also used for antineutrophil cytoplasmic antibodies (ANCA). This is assay to detect autoantibodies directed against antigens found in cytoplasmic granules of neutrophils and monocytes (Van der Woude et al. 1989). ANCAs are closely associated with Wegener granulomatosis, microscopic polyangitis, and Churg–Strauss syndrome (Schmitt and Van der Woude 2004). Determination of ANCA by IIF using neutrophil preparations yields three patterns: cytoplasmic (C-ANCA), perinuclear (P-ANCA) and atypical (A-ANCA) (Savige et al., 1998; Wiik, 2002). C-ANCA is associated with anti-proteinase 3 (PR3) antibodies and P-ANCA with anti-myeloperoxidase (MPO) antibodies. A-ANCA is a perinuclear pattern obtained with ethanol-fixed neutrophils, but negative with formalin-fixed neutrophils. In A-ANCA, the main target antigens are lactoferrin, elastase and cathepsin G. The A-ANCA pattern is mainly observed in non-vasculitic diseases, such as rheumatoid arthritis, intestinal bowel diseases and infectious bacterial or viral diseases (Savige et al. 1998). Other autoantibodies measured by IIF are anti-mitochondrial antibodies (AMA), anti-smooth muscle antibodies, anti-liver and kidney microsomal (LKM) antibodies, antiparietal cell antibodies, anti-adrenal cell antibodies and other organ-specific autoantibodies. The second solution was thought to introduce fully automated IIF interpretation systems with pattern-recognition software. However, as noted above, two of the objections to IIF are its subjectivity and therefore it cannot be completely automated. In contrast some researchers have claimed that this technique is becoming out-of-date and that it should be replaced by enzyme immunoassays or multiplexed assays in the routine laboratory diagnostics (Dahle et al. 2004).

5.5. Detection of Autoantibodies by Proteomic's Technology

Clinical proteomics offers opportunities to identify new disease biomarkers in body fluids, cells and tissues. The focus of clinical proteomics is on the analytical and clinical validation and implementation of novel diagnostic or therapy related markers (Apweiler et al. 2009). Antigen microarrays allow the comprehensive analysis of autoantibodies directed against hundreds to thousands of antigens, including proteins, peptides, nucleic acids, and macromolecular complexes (Joos et al. 2001). Among this future assays are the ***Multiplexed immunoassays***; *Microarray based assays and Flow cytometry*. As yet, arrays for autoantibodies have not been commercialized, but in the coming future this technology should be accessible to clinical autoimmunity laboratories.

5.6. Differences between Laboratory Diagnostic Methods

With the development of new technologies, there is a need to evaluate and standardize the technologies or diagnostic kits in an appropriate clinical laboratory setting (Fritzler, 2006). Many studies conducted under standardized conditions showed the analytical variability of different test systems (Tan 1999). Specificities and sensitivities of autoantibodies against different antigens are important for the diagnosis, but variability in results depend on the source of antigen, assays reproducibility, precision and accuracy and clinical manifestation of diseases (Eissfeller 2005, Törn et al. 2008). Some studies showed agreement between IIF and EIA (Hayashi et al. 2001, Orton et al. 2004) while others demonstrated differences in results (Hoffman et al. 2002, Rouquette and Desgruelles 2006). However, the choice of test is highly dependent on the clinical setting and higher sensitivity and specificity strongly depend on the cut-off value (Hayashi et al. 2001).

Conclusion

In autoimmune diseases, autoantibodies frequently cause tissue injury. This occurs not only by direct activation of effector pathways, but also by uptake and ingestion of immune complexes by cells, leading to cell activation and release of inflammatory cytokines. The specificity of many auto-antibodies has great diagnostic utility and might also have predictive value, such as with anti-CCP autoantibodies in rheumatoid arthritis. The specificity of autoantibodies in autoimmunity suggests an intimate relationship with disease etiology and pathogenesis.

References

Al Jabri AA, Al Buloshi MS. (2004). Anticardiolipin and antinuclear antibodies in the adult healthy Omani individuals. *Saudi. Med. J.* 25(3):313-7.

Al-Jabri AA, Al Belushi MS, Nsanze H. (2003). Frequency and levels of autoantibodies in healthy adult Omanis. *Ann. Saudi. Med.* 23(6):372-5.

Al-Shukaily AA, Al-Jabri AA. (2006) Rheumatoid arthritis, cytokines and hypoxia: what is the link? *Saudi. Medical Journal*, Volume 27(11):447-455.

Amagai, M. (2003). Desmoglein as a target in autoimmunity and infection. J Am Acad Dermatol, 48(2), 244-252.

Apweiler R, Aslandis C, Defuel T, Gerstner A, et al. (2009). Approaching clinical proteomics: current state and future fields of application in fluid proteomics. *Clin. Chem. Lab. Med.* 47, 724-44.

Bahn RS and Heufelder AE. (1993). Pathogenesis of Graves' ophthalmopathy. *N. Engl. J. Med.,* 329(20), 1468-1475.

Barcellos LF, Kamdar BB, Ramsay PP, DeLoa C, Lincoln RR, Caillier S, Schmidt S, Haines JL, Pericak-Vance MA, Oksenberg JR, Hauser SL. (2006). Clustering of autoimmune diseases in families with a high-risk for multiple sclerosis: a descriptive study. *Lancet Neurol.* 5(11):924-31.

Beardsley DS and Ertem M. (1998). Platelet autoantibodies in immune thrombocytopenic purpura. *Transfus. Sci.,* 19(3), 237-244.

Bogdanos DP, Choudhuri K, Vergani D. (2001). Molecular mimicry and autoimmune liver disease: virtuous intentions, malign consequences. Liver 21(4):225-32.

Bossuyt X, Frans J, Hendrickx A, et al. (2004). Detection of Anti-SSA Antibodies by Indirect Immunofluorescence. *Clin. Chem.* 12: 2361-9.

Burlingame RW. (2004). Recent advances in understanding the clinical utility and underlying cause of antinucleosome (antichromatin) autoantibodies. *Clin. Appl. Immunol. Rev.,* 4, 351 – 66.

Clynes R and Ravetch JV. (1995). Cytotoxic antibodies trigger inflammation through Fc receptors. *Immunity*, 3(1), 21-26.

Cross AH, Trotter, JL, et al. (2001). B cells and antibodies in CNS demyelinating disease. *J. Neuroimmunol.*, 112(1-2), 1-14.

Cunningham M, Gilkeson G. (2011). Estrogen receptors in immunity and autoimmunity.*Clin. Rev. Allergy Immunol.* 40(1):66-73.

Cutolo M, Straub RH. (2009). Insights into endocrine-immunological disturbances in autoimmunity and their impact on treatment. *Arthritis Res. Ther.* 11(2):218.

Dahle C, Skogh T, Åberg AK, Jalal A, et al. (2004). Methods of choice for diagnostics antinuclear antibody (ANA) screening: Benefit of adding antigen-specific assays to immunofluorescence microscopy. *J. Autoimmun.,* 22, 241-8.

Damle RN, Fais F, Ghiotto F, Valetto A, Albesiano E, Wasil T, Batliwalla FM, Allen SL, Schulman P, Vinciguerra VP, Rai KR, Gregersen PK, Ferrarini M, Chiorazzi N. (2000). Chronic lymphocytic leukemia: a proliferation of B cells at two distinct stages of differentiation. *Curr. Top Microbiol. Immunol.* 252:285-92.

Domen RE. (1998). An overview of immune hemolytic anemias. *Cleve. Clin. J. Med.,* 65(2), 89-99.

Dörner T, Lipsky PE. (2006). Signalling pathways in B cells: implications for autoimmunity. *Curr. Top Microbiol. Immunol.* 305:213-40.

Eissfeller P, Sticherling M, Scholz D, et al. (2005). Comparison of Different Test Systems for Simultaneous Autoantibody Detection in Connective Tissue Diseases. Ann NY Acad Sci, 1050, 1-13.

Elkon K and Casali P. (2008). Nature and functions of autoantibodies. *Nat. Clin. Pract. Rheumatol.,* 4(9), p491–498.

Felix NJ, Suri A, Salter-Cid L, Nadler SG, Gujrathi S, Corbo M, Aranda R. (2010). Targeting lymphocyte co-stimulation: from bench to bedside. *Autoimmunity*43(7):514-25.

Firestein GS. (2003). Evolving concepts of rheumatoid arthritis. *Nature,* 423(6937), 356-361.

Frisoni L, McPhie L, et al. (2005). Nuclear autoantigen translocation and autoantibody opsonization lead to increased dendritic cell phagocytosis and presentation of nuclear antigens: a novel pathogenic pathway for autoimmunity? *J. Immunol.,* 175(4), 2692-2701.

Fritzler MJ. (2006). Advances and applications of multiplexed diagnostic technologies in autoimmune diseases. *Lupus,* 15, 422-7.

Gaipl US, Munoz LE, et al. (2007). Clearance deficiency and systemic lupus erythematosus (SLE). *J. Autoimmun.*, 28(2-3), 114-121.

Gonza´lez C, Guevara P, Garcı´a-Berrocal B, et al. (2004). Clinical evaluation of Cobas Core anti-dsDNA EIA Quant. *J. Clin. Lab. Anal*, 18, 200– 5.

Gonza´lez-Buitrago J.M, Gonza´lez C, Hernando M, et al. (2003). Antibodies to centromere antigens measured by an automated enzyme immunoassay. *Clin. Chim. Acta*, 328, 135–8.

González-Buitrago JM and González C. (2006). Present and future of the autoimmunity laboratory. *Clin. Chim. Acta*, 365, 50-7.

Green NM, Marshak-Rothstein A. (2011). Toll-like receptor driven B cell activation in the induction of systemic autoimmunity. *Semin. Immunol.* 23(2):106-12.

Hansen A, Dörner T, Lipsky PE. (2000). Use of immunoglobulin variable-region genes by normal subjects and patients with systemic lupus erythematosus. *Int. Arch. Allergy Immunol.* 123(1):36-45.

Hayashi N, Kawamoto T, Mukai M, et al., (2001). Detection of Antinuclear Antibodies by Use of an Enzyme Immunoassay with Nuclear Hep-2 Cell Extract and Recombinant Antigens: Comparison with Immunofluorescence Assay in 307 Patients. *Clin. Chem.*, 47, 1649-59.

Hoffman I.E.A, Peene I, Veys E.M, et al. (2002). Detection of Specific Antinuclear Reactivities in Patients with Negative Anti-nuclear Antibody Immunofluorescence Screening Tests. *Clin. Chem.,* 48, 2171-6.

Holdenrieder S, Eichhorn P, Beuers U, Samtleben W, Schoenermarck U, Zachoval R, Nagel D, Stieber P. (2006). Nucleosomal DNA fragments in autoimmune diseases. *Ann. N. Y. Acad. Sci.* 1075:318-27.

Jaskowski TD, Schroder C, Martins TB, et al. (1996). Screening for antinuclear antibodies by enzyme immunoassay. *Am. J. Clin. Pathol.,* 105, 468-73.

Joos TO, Stoll D, (2001). Templin MF. Miniaturised multiplexed immunoassays. *Curr. Opin. Chem. Biol.,* 6, 76-80.

Kipps TJ, Tomhave E, Pratt LF, Duffy S, Chen PP, Carson DA. (1989). Developmentally restricted immunoglobulin heavy chain variable region gene expressed at high frequency in chronic lymphocytic leukemia. *Proc. Natl. Acad. Sci. USA.* 86(15):5913-7.

Kirtland HH 3rd, Mohler DN, Horwitz DA. (1980). Methyldopa inhibition of suppressor-lymphocyte function: a proposed cause of autoimmune hemolyticanemia. *N. Engl. J. Med.* 302(15):825-32.

Kotzin BL. (1996). Systemic lupus erythematosus. *Cell*, 85(3), 303-306.

Lacroix-Desmazes S, Kaveri SV, Mouthon L, Ayouba A, Malanch`ere E, Coutinho A and Kazatchkine MD. (1998). Self-reactive antibodies_natural autoantibodies in healthy Individuals. *Journal of Immunological Methods*, 216, p117-137.

Liao L, R Sindhwani, M Rojkind, S Factor, L Leinwand, and B Diamond. (1995). Antibody-mediated autoimmune myocarditis depends on genetically determined target organ sensitivity. *J. Exp. Med.* 181(3):1123-31.

Lleo A, Invernizzi P, Gao B, Podda M and Gershwin ME. (2010). Definition of human autoimmunity-autoantibodies versus autoimmune diseases. *Autoimmunity Reviews*, 9, A259-A266.

Lleo A, Selmi C, et al. (2008). The consequences of apoptosis in autoimmunity. *J. Autoimmun.,* 31(3), 257-262.

Malmstrom V, Ho KKY, Lun J, Tam PPL, Cheah KSE and Holmdahl R. (1997). Arthritis susceptibility in mice expressing human type II collagen in cartilage. *Scand. J. Immunol.* 45(6):670-7.

Malmstrom V, Kjellen P and Holmdahl R. (1998). Type II collagen in cartilage evokes peptide-specific tolerance and skews the immune response. J Autoimmun. 11(3):213-21.

Meffre E, Casellas R, Nussenzweig MC. (2000). Antibody regulation of B cell development. *Nat. Immunol.* 1(5):379-85.

Meri S and Jarva H. (1998). Complement regulation. *Vox Sang*, 74 Suppl 2, 291-302.

Meriggioli MN and Sanders DB. (2009). Autoimmune myasthenia gravis: emerging clinical and biological heterogeneity. *Lancet Neurol,* 8(5), 475-490.

Monson NL. (2008). The natural history of B cells. *Curr. Opin. Neurol.* 21Suppl 1:S3-8.

Mountz JD, Wang JH, Xie S, Hsu HC. (2011). Cytokine regulation of B-cell migratory behavior favors formation of germinal centers in autoimmune disease. *Discov. Med.* 11(56):76-85.

Nakagawa H and Komorita N. (1993). Complement component C3-derived neutrophil chemotactic factors purified from exudate of rat carrageenin-induced inflammation. *Biochem. Biophys. Res. Commun.,* 194(3), 1181-1187.

Nescakova Z, Bystricky SB. (2011). Cells - ontogenesis and immune memory development. *Gen. Physiol. Biophys.* 30(1):1-10.

Nimmerjahn F and Ravetch JV. (2006). Fc gamma receptors: old friends and new family members. *Immunity*, 24(1), 19-28.

Nossent H and Rekvig OP. (2001). Antinuclear antibody screening in this new millenium: farewell to the microscope? *Scand. J. Rheumatol.* 30,123–6.

Ooi JD, Holdsworth SR, et al. (2008). Advances in the pathogenesis of Goodpasture's disease: from epitopes to autoantibodies to effector T cells. *J. Autoimmun.*, 31(3), 295-300.

Orton SM, Peace-Brewer A, Schmitz JL, et al. (2004). Practical Evaluation of Methods for Detection and Specificity of Autoantibodies to Extractable Nuclear Antigens. *Clin. Diagn. Lab. Immunol.* 11:297-301.

Racanelli V, Prete M, Musaraj G, Dammacco F, Perosa F. (2011). Autoantibodies to intracellular antigens: Generation and pathogenetic role. *Autoimmun. Rev.* 10(8):503-8.

Rantapaa-Dahlqvist S, de Jong BA, et al. (2003). Antibodies against cyclic citrullinated peptide and IgA rheumatoid factor predict the development of rheumatoid arthritis. *Arthritis Rheum.,* 48(10), 2741-2749.

Ravichandran KS and Lorenz U. (2007). Engulfment of apoptotic cells: signals for a good meal. *Nat. Rev. Immunol.*, 7(12), 964-974.

Rodien P, Madec AM, et al. (1996). Antibody-dependent cell-mediated cytotoxicity in autoimmune thyroid disease: relationship to antithyroperoxidase antibodies. *J. Clin. Endocrinol. Metab.*, 81(7), 2595-2600.

Rouquette AM and Desgruelles C. (2006). Detection of antibodies to dsDNA: an overview of laboratory assays. *Lupus* 15, 403-7.

Sandel PC, Monroe JG. (1999). Negative selection of immature B cells by receptor editing or deletion is determined by site of antigen encounter. *Immunity* 10(3):289-99.

Sauerborn M and Schellekens H. (2009). B-1 cells and naturally occurring antibodies: influencing the immunogenicity of recombinant human therapeutic proteins? *Curr. Opin. Biotechnol.,* 20(6), p715-21.

Schieren G and Hansch GM. (1993). Membrane-associated proteins regulating the complement system: functions and deficiencies. *Int. Rev. Immunol.,* 10(1), 87-101.

Savige JA, Paspaliaris B, Silvestrini R, et al. (1998). A review of immunofluorescence patterns associated with antineutrophil cytoplasmic antibodies (ANCA) and their differentiation from other antibodies. *J. Clin. Pathol.,* 51, 568– 75.

Schelonka RL, Szymanska E, Vale AM, Zhuang Y, Gartland GL, Schroeder HW Jr. (2010). DH and JH usage in murine fetal liver mirrors that of human fetal liver. *Immunogenetics* 62(10):653-66.

Schmitt WH, van der Woude FJ. (2004). Clinical applications of antineutrophil cytoplasmic antibody testing. *Curr. Opin. Rheumatol.,* 16, 9–17.

Shlomchik M, Mascelli M, Shan H, Radic MZ, Pisetsky D, Marshak-Rothstein A, Weigert M. (1990). Anti-DNA antibodies from autoimmune mice arise by clonal expansion and somatic mutation. *J. Exp. Med.* 171(1):265-92.

Shoenfeld Y and Katz U. (2005). IVIg therapy in autoimmunity and related disorders: our experience with a large cohort of patients. *Autoimmunity*, 38(2), 123-137.

Silberstein LE. (1993). Natural and pathologic human autoimmune responses to carbohydrate antigens on red blood cells. *Springer. Semin. Immunopathol.,* 15(2-3), 139-153.

Silveira PA and Grey ST. (2006). B cells in the spotlight: innocent bystanders or major players in the pathogenesis of type 1 diabetes. *Trends. Endocrinol. Metab,* 17(4), 128-135.

Singh RR. (2005). SLE: translating lessons from model systems to human disease. *Trends. Immunol.,* 26(11), 572-579.

Smiley JD, Moore SE Jr. (1988). Molecular mechanisms of autoimmunity. *Am. J. Med. Sci.* 295(5):478-96.

Stinton LM and Fritzler MJ. (2007). A clinical approach to autoantibody testing in systemic autoimmune rheumatic disorders. *Autoimmun. Rev.,* 7:77-84.

Sun J, Fass DN, Hudson JA, Vis MA, et al. (1998). Capture-ELISA based on recombinant proteinase 3 (Pr3) is sensitive for Pr3-ANCA/Pr 3 immune complexes. *J. Immunol. Methods.,* 221, 111 – 23.

Sutton, B, Corper A, et al. (2000). The structure and origin of rheumatoid factors. *Immunol. Today,* 21(4), 177-183.

Tan EM. (1989). Antinuclear antibodies: diagnostic markers for autoimmune diseases and probes for cell biology. *Adv. Immunol.,* 44, 93-151.

Tan EM, Feltkamp TE, Smolen JS, et al. (1997). Range of antinuclear antibodies in ''healthy'' individuals. *Arthritis Rheum.,* 40, 1601–11.

Tan EM, Smolen JS, McDougal JS, et al. (1999). A critical evaluation of enzyme immunoassays for detection of antinuclear autoantibodies of defined specificities. *Arthritis Rheum.,* 42, 455-64.

Tincani A, Andreoli L, Bazzani C, Bosiso D, Sozzani S. (2007). Inflammatory molecules: a target for treatment of systemic autoimmune diseases. *Autoimmun. Rev.* 7(1):1-7.

Törn C, Mueller P, Schlosser M, et al. (2008). Diabetes Antibody Standardization Program: evaluation of assays for autoantibodies to glutamic acid decarboxylase and islet antigen-2. *Diabetologia*, 51, 846-52.

Tzioufas AG, Routsias JG. (2010). Idiotype, anti-idiotype network of autoantibodies: pathogenetic considerations and clinical application. *Autoimmun. Rev.* 9(9):631-3.

Van der Woude FJ, Daha MR, Van Es LA. (1989). The current status of neutrophil cytoplasmic antibodies. *Clin. Exp. Immunol.,* 78, 143– 8.

van Gaalen F, Ioan-Facsinay A, et al. (2005). The devil in the details: the emerging role of anticitrulline autoimmunity in rheumatoid arthritis. *J. Immunol.,* 175(9), 5575-5580.

Vincent A, Lily O, et al. (1999). Pathogenic autoantibodies to neuronal proteins in neurological disorders. *J. Neuroimmunol.,* 100(1-2), 169-180.

Von PAJM, Bast EJEG, Derksen RHWM. (2006). Cost-effective detection of non-antidouble-stranded DNA antinuclear antibody specificities in daily clinical practice. *Reumatology*, 45, 629-35.

Waldner H. (2009). The role of innate immune responses in autoimmune disease development, *Autoimmun. Rev.* 8, p400–404.

Walport MJ. (2001a). Complement. First of two parts. *N. Engl. J. Med.*, 344(14), 1058-1066.

Walport, M. J. (2001b). Complement. Second of two parts. *N. Engl. J. Med.*, 344(15), 1140-1144.

Whittingham S, Mackey IR. (1976). Adverse reactions to drugs: relationship to immunopathic disease. *Med. J. Aust.* 1(14):486-8, 490-2.

Wiik AS. (2005). Anti-nuclear autoantibodies. Clinical utility for diagnosis, prognosis, monitoring, and planing strategy in systemic immunoinflammatory diseases. *Scand. J. Rheumatol.*, 34, 260-8.

Wucherpfennig KW. (2001). Mechanisms for the induction of autoimmunity by infectious agents. *J. Clin. Invest.* 108(8):1097-104.

Yanaba K, Bouaziz JD, et al. (2008). B-lymphocyte contributions to human autoimmune disease. *Immunol. Rev.*, 223, 284-299.

Yarkoni Y, Getahun A, Cambier JC. (2010). Molecular underpinning of B-cell anergy. *Immunol. Rev.* 237(1):249-63.

Yu L and Eisenbarth GS. (2004). Humoral autoimmunity. In: G.S. Eisenbarth (Ed.), *Immunology of Type 1 Diabetes* (2nd edition, pp. 247-260). Ausin, TX: Landes Bioisceince.

In: Autoantibodies
Editors: G. E. Jenkins and J. I. Hall

ISBN: 978-1-62081-560-1

Chapter VII

B CELLS AND AUTOANTIBODIES IN MULTIPLE SCLEROSIS

Klaartje Somers*[*,#], *Judith Fraussen, Myrthe Rouwette, Cindy Govarts, Piet Stinissen and Veerle Somers

Hasselt University, Biomedical Research Institute,
Agoralaan, building C, Belgium

ABSTRACT

During the last decades, investigations into MS have centered predominantly on the pathogenic role of autoreactive T cells rather than B cells. Recently, more evidence for a role of the humoral immune response in the MS pathogenesis is provided by the efficiency of novel treatment strategies; the preliminary positive results of intravenous immunoglobulin (IVIG) and B cell targeting therapy (Rituximab) in a group of MS patients have led to a renewed focus on B cells and autoantibodies in this autoimmune disease. In this chapter, we describe the humoral immune response in MS. The B cell repertoire in healthy individuals and MS patients is discussed. Next, B cell functions in MS as well as B cell migration and survival in the central nervous system (CNS) are outlined. An overview is given of the evidence for the involvement of B cells in the

[*] Corresponding author: Veerle Somers, Hasselt University, Biomedical Research Institute, Agoralaan, building C, 3590 Diepenbeek, Belgium, tel. +3211269202, email: veerle.somers@uhasselt.be

[#] Both authors contributed equally

pathogenesis of MS. Finally, different technologies for the study of the humoral reactivity profile in MS are described, including autoantibody profiling and B cell reactivity analysis. Phage display and B cell immortalization are described in more detail as examples of both reactivity screening approaches. The analysis of the reactivity profile of B cells and autoantibodies in MS is relevant for the identification of novel disease markers for diagnosis, prognosis and theranostics, as well as for the elucidation of the underlying disease processes to discover highly needed novel therapeutic targets for the disease. Multiple sclerosis (MS) has been regarded as a T cell mediated disorder for a long time. This focus on T cells was partly attributed to the long-standing observation that an important lymphocytic subset in MS lesions was composed of T cells [1]. In addition, the clear pathogenic effect of myelin-reactive T cells in the animal model of MS, experimental autoimmune encephalomyelitis (EAE), contributed to the belief that autoreactive T cells were at the center of the MS pathogenic processes [2]. Recent studies into B cell and antibody-depleting therapeutic strategies in MS have renewed interest into the involvement of B cells in the underlying disease pathogenesis [3-6]. During the last decades, more and more evidence has been collected for an important role of the humoral immune response in MS pathogenesis.

In this chapter, the B cell repertoire in healthy individuals and MS patients will first be discussed. Next, B cell functions in MS, B cell migration and survival in the central nervous system (CNS) are outlined. An overview is given of the evidence for the involvement of B cells in the pathogenesis of MS. Finally, different technologies for the study of the humoral reactivity profile in MS are described.

1. The B Cell Repertoire in Healthy Individuals and MS Patients

In order to examine the role of B cells in the pathogenesis of MS, it is important to understand the B cell maturation process. The distribution of the different B cell subpopulations that make up the B cell repertoire in healthy individuals and MS patients has already been thoroughly analyzed.

1.1. B Cell Maturation

Mature naïve B cells, which are characterized by expression of the general B cell marker CD19 and the absence of CD27 and CD38 on their surface [7], are released in the peripheral blood after development in the bone marrow and secondary lymphoid organs [8;9]. Recognition of an antigen in lymphoid tissue triggers B cell activation, which is accompanied by an upregulation of CD80 and CD86 surface expression. After activation, B cells proliferate into plasma blasts that produce low-affinity antibody for a few days [10] or further differentiate into different effector B cell subtypes in germinal centers (GC) via the centrocyte and centroblast stages [11]. This differentiation is accompanied by an upregulation of CD38 surface expression [12-14]. In this case, memory B cells, plasma blasts or plasma cells are developed after extensive mutation and maturation [15; 16]. Memory B cells, expressing both CD19 and the memory surface marker CD27 [7], are able to reactivate and differentiate into plasma cells very fast upon a new challenge with their antigen. Plasma cells have lost proliferating capacity and are mostly long-lived antibody-producing cells that no longer display CD19 but do express CD38, CD138 and CD27. Plasma blasts, on the other hand, are short-lived antibody-secreting cells expressing CD19, CD27, CD38 but also the plasma cell marker CD138.

1.2. B Cell Repertoire in Healthy Individuals and MS Patients

In healthy individuals, most B cells that populate the peripheral blood belong to the naïve B cell population, although some circulating memory B cells can be denoted. The antibody-secreting effector cells move into the target tissues to eliminate their target cells and consequently cannot be found in the blood. B cells are rarely found in the cerebrospinal fluid (CSF) of healthy persons and patients with a non-inflammatory neurological disease (NIND) [16]. The peripheral blood of MS patients displays a similar B cell subtype distribution as that of healthy individuals, mostly harbouring B cells with a $CD19^{+}CD27^{-}$ naïve phenotype [17;18].

The CSF of MS patients and patients with other inflammatory neurological disorders (OIND) contains on average 4-5% of $CD19^{+}$ B cells, opposite to the situation in healthy persons. Variability in CSF B cell numbers was seen between patients [16; 17; 19-21], but the majority were mature $CD19^{+}CD27^{+}CD38^{-}CD138^{-}$ memory B cells [17; 18; 22]. $CD19^{+}CD38^{high}CD77^{+}$ $Ki67^{+}Bcl\text{-}2^{-}$ centroblasts, that normally only occur in GC in lymphatic tissues [23], were demonstrated in the CSF [16;18], either as the result of circulating memory B cell recruitment to the CNS or intrathecal differentiation of naïve B cells.

Table 1. Overview B cell subsets in healthy individuals and MS: expression of surface markers and distribution in periphery and CSF

	naïve B cell	memory B cell	plasma blast	centro blast	plasma cell	references
surface markers	$CD19^+$ $CD27^-$ $CD38^-$	$CD19^+$ $CD27^+$ $CD138^-$ $CD38^-$	$CD19^+$ $CD27^{high}$ $CD138^+$ $CD38^+$	$CD19^+$ $CD77^+$ $Ki67^+$ $Bcl\text{-}2^-$ $CD38^{high}$	$CD19^-$ $CD27^{high}$ $CD138^+$ $CD38^+$	[16-19;25;27]
healthy persons						
periphery	+	(+)	-	-	-	[18;26]
CSF	-	-	-	-	-	[17;20;28]
multiple sclerosis						
periphery	+	(+)	-	-	-	[17;18;20;28]
CSF	-	+	+	+	+/(+)	[16-21;25;28]

+ present; - not present; (+) present in low amounts.

Both processes can be promoted by ectopic GC that were identified in the meninges of MS patients and suggest that antibody-secreting cells can be generated within the CNS [24]. Plasma blasts ($CD19^+CD38^+CD138^+$) have also been described as an important CSF B cell population. Numbers of plasma blasts were significantly increased in CSF of patients with MS and clinically isolated syndrome (CIS), a first (sub) acute neurological event with demyelination, when compared with OIND patients [20]. Furthermore, the number of mature memory B cells and plasma blasts in the CSF of MS patients was correlated with intrathecal immunoglobulin G (IgG) and immunoglobulin M (IgM) production, higher disease activity and lesions on magnetic resonance imaging (MRI), total CSF leukocyte numbers and intrathecal production of MMP-9 (matrix metalloproteinase 9), and the homing chemokine CXCL-13 (chemokine (C-X-C motif) ligand 13) [17; 20]. These findings all indicate that CSF B cells play a role in acute inflammation. Being the most prevalent antibody-secreting cells in the CSF, plasma blasts are held responsible for intrathecal IgG production and are consequently mentioned as main effector B cell population in acute inflammation in MS [17]. Normally, plasma blasts are short-lived antibody-secreting cells that rapidly differentiate into fully mature $CD19^-CD138^+$ plasma cells. In MS, however, plasma blast numbers remained virtually constant over time [17], which might demonstrate an antigen-driven chronic B cell stimulation in the CNS.

Disagreement exists concerning the contribution of $CD19^-CD38^+CD138^+$ plasma cells to the B cell repertoire in the CSF compartment. While some studies pointed out very low numbers of plasma cells [17;20;25], another study demonstrated a high number of plasma cells in the CSF of MS patients [18]. Nevertheless, the distribution of plasma blasts and plasma cells in the CSF remains vague, although $CD19^+CD138^+$ and $CD19^-CD138^+$ cells have recently been shown to be derived from the same progenitor pool and thus represent convergent responses [25]. The absence of plasma cells in the CSF of MS patients in some studies could be explained by the fact that plasma cells migrate to the brain meninges and parenchyma so they are hard to detect in CSF. Moreover, surface marker expression profiles have not been entirely clarified for plasma cells and plasma blasts. Previously, it has even been shown that CD138 was not expressed on the surface of plasma blasts and consequently was the only surface marker allowing to differentiate between plasma cells and plasma blasts [26]. Thus the phenotypic differences between these two cell types still have to be determined in detail. Table 1 gives an overview of the different B cell subsets, their surface marker expression profiles and distribution among peripheral blood and CSF.

2. Functions of B cells in MS Pathogenesis

2.1. Antibody Dependent Functions

B cells in MS have traditionally been associated with the production of autoantibodies. Plasma cells and plasma blasts in the CNS generate antibodies that recognize self antigens. These pathogenic antibodies can clear target cells via antibody-dependent cell-mediated cytotoxicity (ADCC) or complement activation (Figure 1-1) [29-31]. In ADCC, autoantibodies bind Fc receptors on macrophages, neutrophils and natural killer (NK) cells that consequently attack myelin by phagocytosis. This further leads to activation of phagocyte oxidase and secretion of hydrolytic enzymes that induce tissue damage and inflammation [31]. Alternatively, autoantibodies bind directly to their target antigen and activate the complement cascade through complement fixation.

The Fc region of the antibody binds to complement component C1q, resulting in activation of the complement cascade. This ultimately leads to the generation of a membrane attack complex (MAC) that is inserted into the cell membrane of the target cell to cause lysis and cell death [31;32].

2.2. Antibody Independent Functions

B cells exert antibody independent functions in MS pathogenesis as well. B cells secrete proinflammatory cytokines, such as interleukin-6 (IL-6) and tumor necrosis factor (TNF), that enhance tissue damage in the CNS by activation of macrophages and T cells (Figure 1-2) [33]. These cytokines can modulate the migration of dendritic cells and provide feedback stimulatory signals for further B cell activation [30].

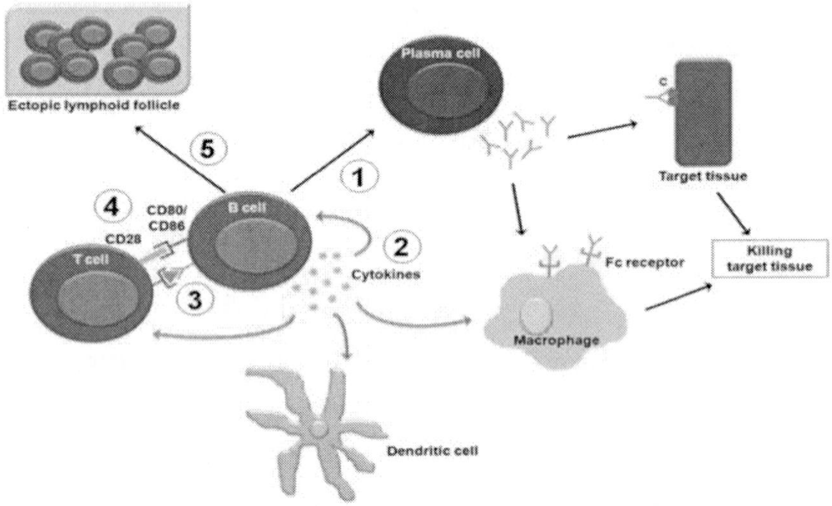

Figure 1. Functions of B cells in MS. (1) Production of (auto)antibodies that cause killing of their target tissue by antibody-dependent cell-mediated cytotoxicity (ADCC) or by complement activation. (2) Secretion of proinflammatory cytokines, such as TNF and IL-6, activate macrophages, T cells and dendritic cells to enhance tissue damage. They also provide positive feedback signals for further B cell activation. Production of IL-10 by B cells causes suppression of the immune response. (3) B cells function as antigen-presenting cells, which results in T cell clonal expansion and cytokine production. (4) B cells provide costimulatory signals during T cell activation. B7 molecules (CD80 or CD86) on B cells bind to CD28 on the T cell surface to provide this costimulation. (5) Formation and maintenance of ectopic GC in the meninges. Abbreviation: c, complement.

The immunosuppressive cytokine interleukin-10 (IL-10) is produced as well, and is more important in dampening of the immune response [16;34]. Although their antigen presenting capacity is low when capturing antigen in a nonspecific manner, B cells are potent antigen-presenting cells (APC) for the activation of T cells of the same specificity [35;36]. In this way, B cells participate in the generation and maintenance of T cell clonal expansion and cytokine production (Figure 1-3).

In addition, B cells provide co-stimulation in the T cell activation process (Figure 1-4) [29;34]. Increase in the number of circulating B cells that express the costimulatory receptors CD80 (cluster of differentiation 80) and CD86 (B7-1) again contributes to T cell clonal expansion and cytokine production [37; 38].

Furthermore, B cells are involved in the formation and maintenance of ectopic lymphoid follicles (Figure 1-5), large B cell aggregates in the meninges of MS patients. The formation of such follicular structures is driven by dendritic cells and B cells through the actions of cytokines and chemokines including CXCL-12, CXCL-13 and lymphotoxin [18].

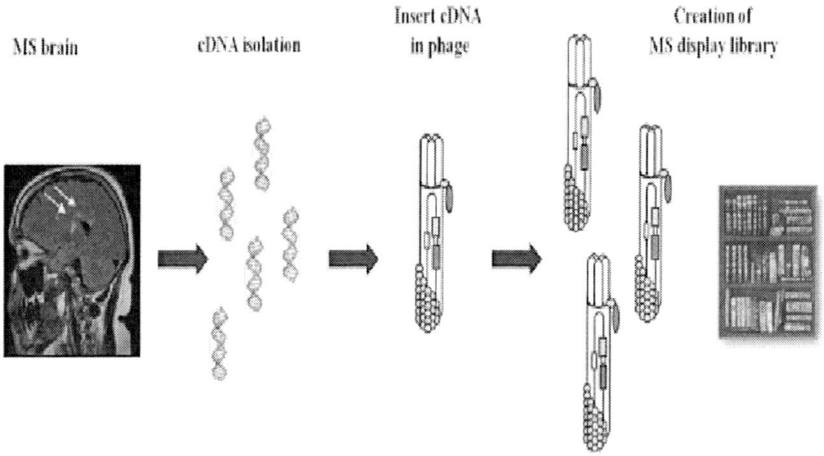

Figure 2. Creation of a cDNA phage display library. The antigenic complexity of diseased tissue is far greater than that of normal tissue. Therefore, MS brain plaques with varying degrees of demyelination and inflammatory activity are used for the construction of the MS cDNA phage display library. cDNA from the MS plaques is isolated and subsequently incorporated in the genome of filamentous bacteriophages. Upon phage virion assembly, the (poly)peptide product, encoded by the inserted cDNA, will be expressed at the phage surface as a fusion product with the phage coat protein. By inserting multiple cDNA products in phages, a diverse cDNA library is created.

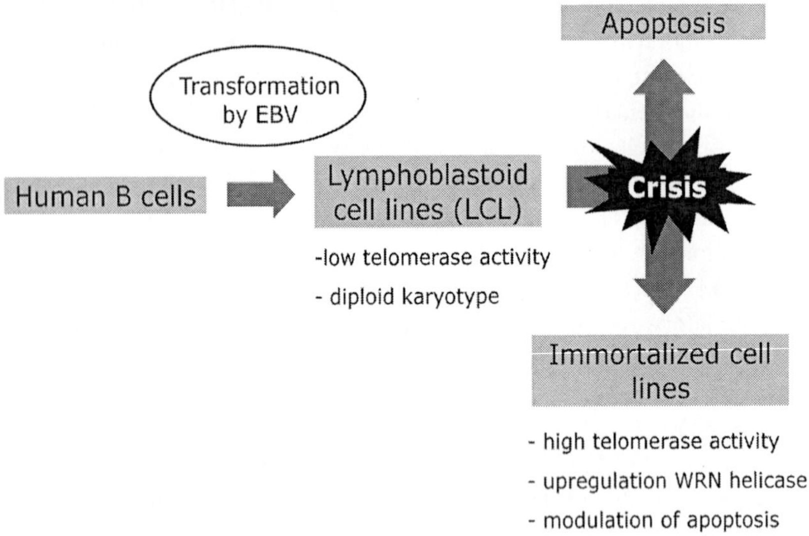

Figure 3. In vitro B cell immortalization process. Human B cells can become infected by EBV and will be transformed into lymphoblastoid cell lines (LCL), characterized by low telomerase activity and normal diploid karyotypes. When telomeres are very short, the transformed B cells go into a proliferative crisis in which most of the cells die because of apoptosis. A small portion of the B cells survive and become immortalized through activation of telomerase. Some other features of immortalized B cells are the upregulation of WRN helicase and modulation of apoptosis.

Finally, B cells in MS produce neurotrophic factors such as nerve growth factor [39], brain-derived neurotrophic factor [40] and neurturin [41]. These might help in restoring CNS integrity.

3. B Cell Migration and Survival in the CNS

Migration of B cells to the brain is directed by CXCL-13, CXCL-10 and CXCL-12 that are secreted by endothelial cells and are upregulated in the brain of MS patients [16;42;43]. In addition, migration is facilitated by very late antigen-4 (VLA-4) and lymphocyte function-associated antigen-1 (LFA-1) [42]. These adhesion molecules bind to vascular cell adhesion molecule-1 (VCAM-1) and intercellular adhesion molecule-1 (ICAM-1) on endothelial cells to direct B cells from the circulation into the CNS. BAFF and A proliferation inducing ligand (APRIL) are two important regulators of B cell survival and activation in the CNS, but also of differentiation, germinal center formation and Ig production [44;45].

Both members of the TNF family are produced by monocytes, macrophages and dendritic cells [30]. Their receptors on the B cell surface are BAFF-receptor (BAFF-R), B cell maturation antigen (BCMA) and transmembrane activator and calcium modulator and cytophilin ligand interactor (TACI) [45].

BAFF may synergize with CXCL-12, CXCL-13 and CCL-19 (chemokine (C-C motif) ligand 19) to attract and maintain B cells in the inflamed CNS of MS patients [46]. Levels of BAFF, BAFF-R and APRIL messenger RNA (mRNA) are increased in patients with MS, where they are produced by astrocytes [47-49]. The group of Serafini recently reported strong BAFF immunoreactivity in infiltrating Epstein-Barr virus (EBV)-infected B cells that were organized in ectopic B cell follicles in the meninges of MS brains [50]. BAFF and APRIL have furthermore been described to be relevant targets for therapy of various autoimmune disorders and could be used in that context since intravenous Ig contains anti-BAFF and anti-APRIL antibodies [15;51].

4. Evidence for a Role of B Cells and Autoantibodies in MS Pathogenesis

The first evidence for the presence of a distorted humoral immune response was already detected a long time ago: oligoclonal immunoglobulin (Ig) bands (OCB) were described by Elvin Kabat in 1948 and by EC Laterre in 1964 as being composed of increased Ig generated by antibody-secreting cells in the CNS, thus indicating an intrathecal Ig production in MS [52;53]. At least 2 OCB are present in the CSF that are not present in the corresponding serum sample [54;55].

Two or more OCB exclusive to the CSF are detected in more than 95% of MS patients [56;57] and presence of OCB even constitutes one of the diagnostic criteria for MS [58]. Analysis of the Ig genes of B cells in the CSF and MS lesions confirmed the presence of an intrathecal, antigen-driven, affinity-matured B cell response [59;60].

In addition, B cells, plasma cells, plasma blasts and myelin-binding antibodies have been reported in MS lesions and MS CSF [61-64]. Pattern II demyelinating lesions, characterized by Ig deposits and involvement of the complement system, are furthermore the most frequent (approximately 58%)

lesion type in MS patients [65]. B cell cytokines, such as BAFF (B cell activating factor of the TNF family, tumor necrosis factor ligand superfamily member 13B), were also detected in MS lesions [47]. Ectopic lymphoid follicles containing proliferating B cells and plasma cells have recently been demonstrated in the meninges of a subset of MS patients [66;67].

These are large B cell aggregates consisting primarily of memory B cells that are localized in the sub-arachnoid space, mainly inside the cerebral sulci and display several features of germinal centers including the presence of dendritic cells expressing CXCL13, B cell proliferation, expression of activation-induced cytidine deaminase and plasma cell differentiation [68]. Ectopic lymphoid follicles have also been denoted in EAE [69]. Moreover, the presence of a distorted humoral immune response in MS was shown to be associated with a worse disease outcome [70], while findings in EAE supported an important role of the humoral autoimmune response in disease pathology. Passive antibody transfer experiments with antibodies directed against myelin oligodendrocyte glycoprotein (MOG) at the onset of acute EAE in rat resulted in extensive plaque-like demyelination and exacerbation of the clinical signs [71].

For the first time, this study provided clear evidence for the demyelinating capacity of antibodies. Subsequent studies showed that antibodies directed against other prevalent myelin components such as myelin basic protein (MBP) and galactocerebroside (Galc) or neuronal components such as neurofascin also could have an effect on the EAE disease course [72;73]. Besides the role of CNS-reactive antibodies in EAE, B cells have been shown to be required for disease induction in several EAE models (reviewed in [74]).

Recently, more conclusive evidence for a role of the humoral immune response in MS pathogenesis has been provided by the efficiency of novel treatment strategies; the preliminary positive results of intravenous immunoglobulin (IVIG) and B cell depleting therapy (Rituximab) in a group of MS patients have led to a renewed focus on B cells and autoantibodies in this autoimmune disease [75-77].

On the other hand, besides evidence for a pathogenic role of the humoral immune response in MS, there are also indications that B cell cytokines, neurotrophic factors and antibodies might downregulate immune responses and promote repair and remyelination. These findings point towards a beneficial effect of the humoral immune response in the MS disease process [78-80].

The above findings support an important role of B cells in MS. Whether B cells are implicated in disease initiation or whether their involvement is secondary to the causative immune response is still not clear (reviewed in [81]). Further analysis of the antigen reactivity of B cells in MS is warranted to obtain more information regarding the underlying disease processes.

5. Analysis of the Humoral Reactivity Profile in MS

Numerous approaches are currently used to investigate reactivity of the humoral immune response with different success rates, and despite a lot of effort the targets of the autoreactive B cells and antibodies are not yet known. Since MS is characterized by a heterogeneous disease course and genetic background, novel markers for the diagnosis of patients and a multiplex treatment strategy are needed for better control of the disease. Studying the humoral immune response thus remains a hot topic in MS research where identification of the target antigens is one of the main goals.

Different approaches for reactivity analysis of the humoral immune response in MS are discussed below. Phage display and B cell immortalization technology are described in more detail.

CSF can be a useful surrogate for the brain microenvironment and is therefore suitable to study antibody responses in MS. Moreover, oligoclonal Ig have mainly been described in the CSF of MS patients. However, CSF may also comprise antibodies originating from the peripheral blood that are not specific to the disease.

Disease-relevant autoreactive antibodies may even bind to their targets or to Fc receptors in the CNS tissue, rendering them undetectable in CSF. Serum can be used as an alternative to study B cell reactivity in MS. Intrathecally produced antibodies are able to diffuse from the CSF into the circulation, leaving them detectable in the serum. In addition, several studies have described the increased presence of specific antibody reactivity in serum of MS patients when compared to neurological controls, demonstrating that serum autoantibody profiles can be used to distinguish MS patients from control subjects [82-84].

Most studies investigating the specificity of the humoral immune response have focused on autoantibodies directly by analyzing reactivity of the antibodies in serum or CSF of MS patients versus healthy controls or other neurological control patients.

A substantial amount of the already identified candidate autoantigens have been denoted in this way. An alternative approach that does not suffer from binding of antibodies to their target antigens or from dilution and breakdown of antibodies, would be to investigate the reactivity of the expanded (autoreactive) B cells in MS. The main findings of both reactivity profiling approaches in MS are described below.

5.1. Autoantibody Profiling in MS

In the past, different experimental approaches have been used for analysis of the autoantibody specificities in the serum and CSF of MS patients. Table 2 contains a summary of all previously reported antigenic targets of autoantibodies in MS (reviewed in [85;86]). As it is thought that in MS, the myelin in the CNS is the primary target of the aberrant autoimmune response, different myelin components were firstly proposed as candidate autoantigens (Table 2). There are numerous reports about antibodies directed against MBP [87], MOG [88], proteolipid protein (PLP) [89] and myelin-associated glycoprotein (MAG) [90] in MS patients but up till now, none of these myelin-associated candidate antigens definitely discriminates between the humoral immune response in MS patients and healthy controls [91-94]. The true relevance of anti-myelin antibodies in the MS disease process and in the development of MS disease markers remains inconclusive. Moreover, other CNS-specific components such as neuronal, axonal and glial compounds have been analyzed as autoantibody targets in MS (Table 2) [95;96]. There are however also reports about the presence of antibodies against more ubiquitous *self*-antigens such as heat-shock proteins (hsp) [97] and DNA (deoxyribonucleic acid) [98] (Table 2). Up till now, the reported sensitivities and specificities of the identified individual autoantibodies for MS are at best only moderate. Not one of the autoantibodies is specifically present only in MS patients. Moreover, all autoantibodies are present in a subpopulation of MS patients. This can be explained by the enormous heterogeneity which is characteristic for MS and is reflected in the diversity of MS disease courses, treatment efficiencies and prevailing pathogenic processes.

5.1.1. Multiplexing Approaches for Autoantibody Profiling in MS

In recent years, the need for multiplex autoantibody profiling approaches has become evident within the research domain of autoimmunity [99; 100], since autoimmune diseases are characterized by broad autoantibody profiles with considerable overlap between the different diseases [101;102]. This overlap in reactivity profile and the heterogeneous nature of MS, represented in the diversity of disease courses, treatment efficiencies and prevailing pathogenic processes, underscore the importance of a multiplexing approach to fully elucidate the MS autoantibody profile.

The identification of a MS-specific autoantibody fingerprint can be of great use from a diagnostic point of view, but can also provide valuable information regarding disease-specific humoral immune responses and thus the underlying autoimmune aetiology and pathogenesis. Different multiplexing approaches such as the use of antigen microarrays, high-throughput blotting procedures and lambda phage expression library screening, have already been used for the identification of a disease-specific autoantibody fingerprint in MS serum and MS CSF.

By application of lipid-antigen microarrays for autoantibody profiling in MS CSF, Kanter *et al.* demonstrated increased lipid-specific antibody reactivity against different myelin lipids including sulfatide, sphingomyelin, oxidized lipids and microbial lipids in individuals with MS [103]. Based on a similar microarray technology, Quintana *et al.* recently reported the identification of unique serum autoantibody patterns that distinguished relapsing-remitting MS (RRMS), secondary progressive MS (SPMS) and primary progressive MS (PPMS) patients from each other and from healthy controls (HC) and patients with other neurological and autoimmune diseases [104]. Moreover, patients with different immunopathologic patterns of MS (based on brain biopsy analysis) could be discerned based on unique autoantibody profiles [105].

However, despite the interesting results obtained, the main drawback of antigen array screening is the fact that it is a so-called biased autoantibody profiling approach; only a small number of known and characterized antigens are spotted as candidate antigenic targets, which is not fully representative for the heterogeneity present within the *in vivo* target tissue in MS, namely the inflamed CNS. Moreover, by applying this approach, the identification of novel antigenic targets is not possible.

An alternative, less biased protein array system for autoantibody profiling in MS was applied by the research group of Hemmer [106]. Protein arrays were prepared by the spotting of 37,000 different expression clones, obtained from a human fetal brain complementary DNA (cDNA) library. Probing of these arrays with individual CSF samples from MS and control patients resulted in the identification of two EBV proteins (Table 2) against which significantly higher serum and CSF immunoreactivities were identified in MS patients [107].

Table 2. MS antibody reactivities

Myelin antigens (proteins, glycoproteins and lipids)		
	Myelin oligodendrocyte glycoprotein	[115]
	Myelin basic protein	[116;117]
	Myelin associated glycoprotein	[118]
	Proteolipid protein	[119]
	CSF114(Glc)	[120]
	Glc(alpha1,4)Glc(alpha)	[121]
	Myelin lipids (phosphatidylcholine, sulfatide, sphingomyelin)	[122;123]
	Galactocerebroside	[124]
	Cerebellar soluble lectin	[125]
Axonal and neuronal antigens		
	Neurofilaments (light and medium chain)	[126]
	Gangliosides (GD1a, GM3, sulfatide)	[127]
	Axolemma-Enriched Fraction	[128]
	Tubulin	[129]
	Nogo-A	[130]
	Nogo receptor	[131]
	Surface antigen on neuronal cell line	[132]
	Neurofascin 186	[133]
	Contactin-2	[134]
Oligodendrocyte antigens		
	Surface antigen on oligodendrocyte-precursor derived cell line	[135]
	Oligodendrocyte progenitor cell-specific surface glycoprotein	[136]
	Oligodendrocyte-specific protein	[137]
	Transaldolase	[138]
	2',3'-cyclic nucleotide 3' phosphodiesterase	[139]
Stress proteins		
	Alpha-B-crystallin	[140]
	Hsp60	[141]
	Hsp70	[142]
	Hsp90β	[143]
Ubiquitous and other antigens		
	Proteasome	[144]
	DNA	[145]

	Heterogeneous nuclear ribonucleoprotein B1	[146]
	Retinal arrestin	[147]
	Triosephosphate isomerase	[148]
	Glyceraldehyde 3-phosphate dehydrogenase	[149]
	Alu-peptide	[150]
	Epstein-Barr nuclear antigen 1	[151]
	BRRF2 (EBV protein)	[152]

Based on [153;154].

Several research groups have applied more unbiased proteomics approaches to elucidate MS autoantibody profiles. Lefranc *et al.* identified distinct serum IgG antibody repertoires against human brain homogenates between MS patients and control subjects by application of 1-D (1 dimensional) and 2-D (2 dimensional) immunoblotting techniques [108]. Furthermore, specific IgG reactivity profiles that could discriminate between the three forms of MS (RR, SP and PP) were detected [109]. An analogous 1-D immunoblotting procedure of human brain lysates with purified MS CSF IgG by Kolln *et al.* led to the identification of triosephosphate isomerase (TPI) and glyceraldehyde 3-phosphate dehydrogenase (GAPDH) as MS CSF antibody targets (Table 2) [110]. A similar proteomics approach was applied by the research groups of Linington and Meinl. In this study, serum and Ig preparations from MS and control patients were used in 1-D and 2-D blotting experiments of glycoproteins isolated from human myelin by lentil-lectin affinity chromatography [111;112]. These experiments led to the identification of 2 novel and promising antibody-targets in MS patients, namely neurofascin and contactin-2 (Table 2) [113;114].

The application of immunoblotting of brain preparations for autoantibody profiling allows the identification of novel antigenic targets. In addition, the *in vivo* antigenic composition of the diseased tissue is conserved to a higher extent in this immunoblotting procedure. Drawbacks of the technology are the relatively low sensitivity (especially for less abundant proteins) and the inherent biases in antigen representation due to use of denaturing polyacrylamide gel electrophoresis.

Archelos *et al.* compared pooled CSF from MS patients with that from patients with other neurological diseases by applying a high-throughput filter screening procedure on a lambda phage cDNA expression library constructed from an oligodendrocyte-precursor cell [155]. A sequence motif of 7 amino acids that was homologous to a translated consensus Alu repeat epitope was detected and further analysis showed that 44% of MS sera and CSF reacted with these Alu-peptides (Table 1.1) [156].

Similar screenings of lambda phage expression libraries constructed from chronic MS plaques with MS CSF and MS serum by Owens *et al.* did not result in the identification of MS-specific target antigens [157].

5.1.2. Autoantibody Profiling with Phage Display Technology

More than 20 years ago, phage display technology using filamentous phage was developed by Smith [158]. The technique is based on the ability of phage virions, virus particles that infect and amplify in bacteria, to incorporate foreign DNA into their genome, coupled to a gene encoding a phage coat protein [159;160]. After infection, phage protein components are produced by the protein translation machinery of the infected bacterial host cell and the incorporated DNA is translated into the corresponding DNA product, covalently coupled to the phage coat protein. Upon phage virion assembly, the recombinant coat protein will be incorporated into the virion protein coat [160].

The (poly) peptide product, encoded by the DNA insert, is displayed at the surface of the phage particle and is thus available for experimental strategies. The strength of the phage display technology lies within the physical link between DNA and DNA product (through the protein coat of the virus), which allows for the succession of affinity selection and amplification of selected phage particles resulting in powerful enrichment of selected phage and an increase in assay sensitivity [160;161]. This link between *genotype* and *phenotype* is absent in lambda phage expression library screening assays used to identify ligands for different targets [162;163]. These assays are more labour-intensive and are characterized by lower sensitivities due to the preclusion of phage enrichment.

A commonly used phage display procedure encompasses the display of synthetically produced peptide libraries [164]. This peptide phage display technique has already been applied by several research groups for autoantibody profiling in MS and RA.

The peptide phage display technique was applied by Cortese *et al.* to identify peptide motifs that were recognized by antibodies in the CSF from MS patients. The authors showed that selection with individual MS CSF led to the identification of patient-specific epitopes. Moreover, antibodies against the selected epitopes were demonstrated with a similar frequency in MS sera as compared to control sera [165]. In a new attempt to identify MS-specific epitopes, 20 different MS CSF samples were pooled for selection of a random peptide library, confirming the earlier finding of patient-specific antibody reactivities. The authors concluded that common antibody specificities are absent in MS patients, or that they are present in very low concentrations [166].

However, other research groups who adopted similar peptide phage display strategies for autoantibody profiling in MS were successful at identifying MS-associated peptide motifs. A similar peptide phage display approach was applied by Dybwad *et al.*, who analyzed the CSF antibody specificities within an oligoclonal band from one MS patient using different phage displayed random peptide libraries.

Distinct but structurally related peptide motifs were detected, which showed significant linear homology with collagen proteins, the 68 kDa neurofilament protein, versican and other proteins from viruses such as human cytomegalovirus, herpes simplex virus and human papillomavirus [167].

Jolivet-Reynaud *et al.* reported the use of a decapeptide phage display library to analyze the antibody specificities in the CSF and serum from 4 MS patients. The peptides that were identified by selections with MS serum were not disease-specific while selections performed with CSF resulted in the identification of several motifs which were recognized more specifically in MS CSF compared to CSF from patients with other neurological diseases. Amino acid similarities were detected between the selected peptides and envelope regions of MS-associated retrovirus and the related endogenous retrovirus (HERV-W) [168]. Rand *et al.* have used individual CSF from 14 MS patients for the screening of a hexamer peptide phage display library.

A common motif was selected, which was found in EBV protein EBNA1, alpha B crystalline and in the 65 kDa non-structural cytomegalovirus antigen. It was shown that 60-65% of EBV-seropositive MS patients presented with antibodies against the selected motif [169;170]. The main drawback of the peptide phage display approach is the identification of so-called mimotopes [171].

Mimotopes are peptides forming epitopes that structurally mimic the actual *in vivo* antigens. This implies that the mimotope and the corresponding actual antigen are not necessarily identical or similar at amino acid level, although sequence similarity is not excluded. The identification of the actual *in vivo* antigen of the detected autoantibody requires a labour-intensive and difficult characterization of the identified epitope [172]. This drawback of peptide phage display can partially be overcome by application of cDNA phage display [173]. cDNA phage display entails the display of an entire cDNA expression library allowing interaction between cDNA encoded peptides and proteins exposed on the surface of the phage and antibody selectors. An expression library can be conveniently constructed from cell lines and cell cultures. cDNA phage display of an expression library made from diseased target tissue is even more interesting. The use of affected tissue allows the display of the entire heterogeneous antigen composition within the diseased tissue.

We have developed and used a powerful molecular multiplexing procedure called serological antigen selection (SAS) of which the strength lies within the application of cDNA phage display. Application of the procedure for MS CSF entailed filamentous phage display of a normalized expression library made from three active chronic MS plaques with varying degrees of demyelination and inflammatory activity, obtained from one MS patient (Figure 2) [174].

By using a cDNA expression library from diseased tissue for phage display library construction, the entire heterogeneity of known and novel expressed antigens present within the affected tissue can be displayed and potentially selected.

The antigenic complexity held within the diseased tissue is far greater than that from normal tissue, due to the diversity of processes occurring at this site of autoimmune attack such as inflammatory cell infiltration, activation and migration as well as destruction and possible repair of endogenous tissue cells. Sequencing of the MS cDNA library confirmed the value of the use of a cDNA expression library made from diseased tissue for the identification of autoantibody targets in MS [175].

The percentage of novel genes and the number of expressed sequences were significantly higher in the MS library compared to normal human brain libraries. The detected sequences were associated with the diversity of processes occurring in and around MS lesions such as inflammatory cell infiltration, activation and migration, antigen presentation and tissue damage [176].

By application of affinity selections on the MS cDNA phage display library with pooled CSF from 10 RRMS patients, we recently identified a panel of 4 MS-specific and 4 MS-associated antigenic targets [177]. Immunoreactivity against this panel of 8 novel MS-candidate antigens was analyzed in 73 MS patients, 64 patients with non-inflammatory neurological diseases and 30 patients with other inflammatory neurological diseases.

The sensitivity and specificity values of the detection of antibodies against this panel of 8 autoantibody targets for MS were 45% and 86%, respectively

[178]. Further research is needed to evaluate the biological role of these antigenic targets in the disease process of MS.

5.2. B Cell Reactivity Analysis in MS

Instead of focusing on autoantibody profiling, some studies have analyzed the reactivity of the clonally expanded B cells and plasma cells in the CSF and/or peripheral blood of MS patients. The group of Link *et al.* performed different studies on B cell reactivity in MS using an immunospot assay. Nitrocellulose microtiter plates were coated with myelin antigens to detect binding of peripheral blood mononuclear cells (PBMC) or CSF cells. When studying CSF cells and PBMC of 19 MS patients, MBP-reactive CSF B cells were found in 57% of MS patients while none were present in peripheral blood. MAG-reactive B cells were indicated both in CSF and PBMC of MS patients (55% and 11% of patients, respectively) [179]. Furthermore, anti-MOG IgG secreting cells were demonstrated in PBMC from 8 of 16 MS patients and in CSF from 8 of 10 MS patients [180].

Other studies made use of recombinant antibodies that were produced from patients' B cells. $CD19^+$ or $CD138^+$ cells from CSF were single-cell sorted into PCR plates, the variable regions of the heavy and light Ig chains (V_H and V_L) were amplified and cloned into a plasmid vector which was then expressed in a bacterial expression system.

The corresponding recombinant antibodies were used for reactivity screenings with immunoprecipitation, Western blot, ELISA or immunohistochemistry. Lambracht-Washington and coworkers discovered reactivity of their recombinantly produced antibodies towards MBP, 2',3'-cyclic nucleotide 3'-phosphodiesterase (CNPase) and GFAP [181]. On the other hand, von Büdingen *et al.* produced 9 recombinant MS antibodies following the same procedure, and in this case 8 displayed myelin reactivity and 1 was directed against astroglia [182].

Apart from myelin binding in MS brain tissue, their targets could not be identified using several techniques such as costaining with known myelin antigens on brain tissue in immunohistochemistry, Western blot with human myelin or ELISA using recombinant and native MOG and MBP. In yet another study from Zhang *et al.*, recombinant antibodies from MS CSF demonstrated reactivity to axons with pathologic changes in MS brain tissue [183]. The targets were later identified as TPI and GAPDH [184]. Very recently, Yu *et al.* employed 19 recombinant antibodies from clonally expanded plasma cells in the CSF of MS patients in combination with phage displayed random peptide libraries to demonstrate peptide reactivity[185]. Several antigenic candidates were identified, including stress proteins, cell surface proteins and neuronal proteins.

Another possibility for determination of the B cell target antigens and characterization of the B cell repertoire is the immortalization of B cells from MS patients. Using this technique immortalized B cell clones, that show continuous antibody production, are generated. The target antigens of the produced antibodies can be determined and the B cell response that is going on in vivo can be studied.

5.2.1. B Cell Immortalization

B cell immortalization by EBV has been widely used in immunological, molecular and genetic research as it provides high amounts of DNA and large numbers of B cells and antibody molecules. EBV infects B cells via their CD21 receptor [186] and subsequently transforms them into continually dividing, lymphoblastoid cell lines. Its advantage over other monoclonal antibody producing technologies is the generation of antibodies that represent both the specificity and diversity of the humoral immune response in vivo. Consequently, antibodies produced by B cell immortalization can be useful in several settings in which humoral immunity is involved. Antibodies can even be generated against an infectious agent or tumour cells, rendering these antibodies attractive for therapy.

In vitro infection of B cells from human peripheral blood by EBV causes a transformation into actively proliferating lymphoblastoid cell lines (LCL) [187]. The continuous proliferation of these LCL may be the consequence of the absence of a GC environment where EBNA2, 3A, 3B, 3C and LP are normally downregulated [188]. Shortening of the telomeres occurs because of fast cell division, until the transformed cells go into a proliferative crisis [189]. At this point little or no telomeric DNA remains, leading to apoptosis of a large proportion of the LCL [190]. A small proportion of the transformed cells survive the proliferative crisis through activation of telomerase, the enzyme that elongates telomeres de novo (Figure 3) [191-193].

They become truly immortalized B cell lines that are characterized by downregulation of p16/Rb [187], mutation of the p53 gene [194], modulation of apoptosis [190], upregulation of WRN helicase [194;195], chromosomal instability [194] and a change in cytotoxicity to various chemical compounds [196]. All these features contribute to the evasion of cell death and continuous cell growth.

We have developed an improved B cell immortalization method that is characterized by immortalization efficiencies up to 83% for the generation of IgG-producing immortalized B cell lines from the peripheral blood [197]. Moreover, almost 90% of the produced immortalized B cell lines appeared to be monoclonal, which eliminated the need for subcloning.

For the first time, a B cell immortalization procedure was introduced with high efficiency and reproducibility for low B cell numbers that made immediate generation of monoclonal antibodies, representing the in vivo humoral immune response, possible.

5.2.2. Application of B Cell Immortalization in MS Reactivity Profiling

Using this optimized B cell immortalization method, we have already been able to produce a large panel of immortalized B cell lines from the peripheral blood of MS patients and clinically isolated syndrome (CIS) patients that experienced a first clinical manifestation of MS-like disease [198;199]. Some B cell lines could also be recovered from the CSF of a MS patient. Intracellular autoreactivity of a proportion of the generated immortalized B cell lines from the peripheral blood was demonstrated by analysis of antibody binding to a human oligodendroglioma (HOG) cell line, PBMC and a control human alveolar epithelial (A549) cell line. Further, the immortalized cultures were successfully used for molecular analysis of the Ig heavy chain genes of peripheral and intrathecal B cells. A restricted antigen-stimulated clonally expanded B cell response with possible affinity maturation was hereby demonstrated, not only in CSF but also in peripheral blood of MS and CIS patients (unpublished results). In addition, autoreactivity against striated muscle proteins was shown for immortalized B cell lines that were recovered from MG patients using the same immortalization procedure [200].

These data show how autoreactive antibodies can be produced from patients with autoimmune disease using B cell immortalization. Characterization of these antibodies and identification of the target antigens of these clonally expanded B cells could provide more insight into their relevance in the disease process but could also lead to the identification of novel antigenic targets in MS.

CONCLUSION

Due to the preliminary positive effect of B cell depletion therapy in MS patients, there is renewed interest in the role of autoreactive B cells and autoantibodies in the disease process of multiple sclerosis. Reactivity analysis of the humoral immune response through investigation of autoantibody profiles and B cell reactivity resulted in the identification of a wide range of different B cell and autoantibody targets in MS patients.

However, despite the advances in the knowledge on the humoral reactivity profile in MS patients, up till now, not one autoreactivity was specifically associated with MS. Also, none of the detected autoreactivities was detected in all MS patients. These findings point towards the presence of different autoreactivity profiles in different MS patients, exemplified by the characteristic heterogeneity of the disease. The use of new, highly sensitive and preferably multiplexing technologies such as SAS and EBV B cell immortalization in reactivity analysis can be valuable to expand our current knowledge on the humoral reactivity profile in MS patients.

The elucidation of the MS-associated autoreactivity profile is valuable from a diagnostic biomarker point of view. In addition, the discovery of novel targets of the humoral autoimmune response in MS patients will generate valuable knowledge regarding underlying disease processes and etiology of MS, and can lead to the identification of highly needed, novel therapeutic targets.

References

[1] Traugott U, Reinherz EL, Raine CS. Multiple sclerosis. Distribution of T cells, T cell subsets and Ia-positive macrophages in lesions of different ages. *J. Neuroimmunol.* 1983; 4(3):201-221.

[2] Zamvil SS, Steinman L. The T lymphocyte in experimental allergic encephalomyelitis. *Annu. Rev. Immunol.* 1990; 8:579-621.

[3] Bar-Or A, Calabresi PA, Arnold D, Markowitz C, Shafer S, Kasper LH, Waubant E, Gazda S, Fox RJ, Panzara M, Sarkar N, Agarwal S, Smith CH. Rituximab in relapsing-remitting multiple sclerosis: a 72-week, open-label, phase I trial. *Ann. Neurol.* 2008; 63(3):395-400.

[4] Stuve O, Leussink VI, Frohlich R, Hemmer B, Hartung HP, Menge T, Kieseier BC. Long-term B-lymphocyte depletion with rituximab in patients with relapsing-remitting multiple sclerosis. *Arch. Neurol.* 2009; 66(2):259-261.

[5] Naismith RT, Piccio L, Lyons JA, Lauber J, Tutlam NT, Parks BJ, Trinkaus K, Song SK, Cross AH. Rituximab add-on therapy for

breakthrough relapsing multiple sclerosis: a 52-week phase II trial. *Neurology* 2010; 74(23):1860-1867.

[6] Hauser SL, Waubant E, Arnold DL, Vollmer T, Antel J, Fox RJ, Bar-Or A, Panzara M, Sarkar N, Agarwal S, Langer-Gould A, Smith CH. B-cell depletion with rituximab in relapsing-remitting multiple sclerosis. *N. Engl. J. Med.* 2008; 358(7):676-688.

[7] Klein U, Rajewsky K, Kuppers R. Human immunoglobulin (Ig)M+IgD+ peripheral blood B cells expressing the CD27 cell surface antigen carry somatically mutated variable region genes: CD27 as a general marker for somatically mutated (memory) B cells. *J. Exp. Med.* 1998; 188(9):1679-1689.

[8] Blink E J, Light A, Kallies A, Nutt SL, Hodgkin PD, Tarlinton DM. Early appearance of germinal center-derived memory B cells and plasma cells in blood after primary immunization. *J. Exp. Med.* 2005; 201(4):545-554.

[9] Loken MR, Shah VO, Dattilio KL, Civin CI. Flow cytometric analysis of human bone marrow. II. Normal B lymphocyte development. *Blood* 1987; 70(5):1316-1324.

[10] Ochsenbein AF, Pinschewer DD, Sierro S, Horvath E, Hengartner H, Zinkernagel RM. Protective long-term antibody memory by antigen-driven and T help-dependent differentiation of long-lived memory B cells to short-lived plasma cells independent of secondary lymphoid organs. *Proc. Natl. Acad. Sci. USA* 2000; 97(24):13263-13268.

[11] Klein U, Tu Y, Stolovitzky GA, Keller JL, Haddad J, Jr., Miljkovic V, Cattoretti G, Califano A, Dalla-Favera R. Transcriptional analysis of the B cell germinal center reaction. *Proc. Natl. Acad. Sci. USA* 2003; 100(5):2639-2644.

[12] Dorner T, Radbruch A. Selecting B cells and plasma cells to memory. *J. Exp. Med.* 2005; 201(4):497-499.

[13] Berek C, Berger A, Apel M. Maturation of the immune response in germinal centers. *Cell* 1991; 67(6):1121-1129.

[14] MacLennan IC. Germinal centers. *Annu. Rev. Immunol.* 1994; 12:117-139.

[15] Le Pottier L, Devauchelle V, Pers JO, Jamin C, Youinou P. The mosaic of B-cell subsets (with special emphasis on primary Sjogren's syndrome). *Autoimmun. Rev.* 2007; 6(3):149-154.

[16] Meinl E, Krumbholz M, Hohlfeld R. B lineage cells in the inflammatory central nervous system environment: migration, maintenance, local

antibody production, and therapeutic modulation. *Ann. Neurol.* 2006; 59(6):880-892.

[17] Cepok S, Rosche B, Grummel V, Vogel F, Zhou D, Sayn J, Sommer N, Hartung HP, Hemmer B. Short-lived plasma blasts are the main B cell effector subset during the course of multiple sclerosis. *Brain* 2005; 128(Pt 7):1667-1676.

[18] Corcione A, Casazza S, Ferretti E, Giunti D, Zappia E, Pistorio A, Gambini C, Mancardi GL, Uccelli A, Pistoia V. Recapitulation of B cell differentiation in the central nervous system of patients with multiple sclerosis. *Proc. Natl. Acad. Sci. USA* 2004; 101(30):11064-11069.

[19] Corcione A, Aloisi F, Serafini B, Capello E, Mancardi GL, Pistoia V, Uccelli A. B-cell differentiation in the CNS of patients with multiple sclerosis. *Autoimmun. Rev.* 2005; 4(8):549-554.

[20] Kuenz B, Lutterotti A, Ehling R, Gneiss C, Haemmerle M, Rainer C, Deisenhammer F, Schocke M, Berger T, Reindl M. Cerebrospinal fluid B cells correlate with early brain inflammation in multiple sclerosis. *PLoS ONE* 2008; 3(7):e2559.

[21] Ritchie AM, Gilden DH, Williamson RA, Burgoon MP, Yu X, Helm K, Corboy JR, Owens GP. Comparative analysis of the CD19+ and CD138+ cell antibody repertoires in the cerebrospinal fluid of patients with multiple sclerosis. *J. Immunol.* 2004; 173(1):649-656.

[22] Cepok S, von Geldern G, Grummel V, Hochgesand S, Celik H, Hartung H, Hemmer B. Accumulation of class switched IgD-IgM- memory B cells in the cerebrospinal fluid during neuroinflammation. *J. Neuroimmunol.* 2006; 180(1-2):33-39.

[23] Pascual V, Liu YJ, Magalski A, de Bouteiller O, Banchereau J, Capra JD. Analysis of somatic mutation in five B cell subsets of human tonsil. *J. Exp. Med.* 1994; 180(1):329-339.

[24] Serafini B, Rosicarelli B, Magliozzi R, Stigliano E, Aloisi F. Detection of ectopic B-cell follicles with germinal centers in the meninges of patients with secondary progressive multiple sclerosis. *Brain Pathol.* 2004; 14(2):164-174.

[25] Winges KM, Gilden DH, Bennett JL, Yu X, Ritchie AM, Owens GP. Analysis of multiple sclerosis cerebrospinal fluid reveals a continuum of clonally related antibody-secreting cells that are predominantly plasma blasts. *J. Neuroimmunol.* 2007; 192(1-2):226-234.

[26] Jego G, Robillard N, Puthier D, Amiot M, Accard F, Pineau D, Harousseau JL, Bataille R, Pellat-Deceunynck C. Reactive

plasmacytoses are expansions of plasmablasts retaining the capacity to differentiate into plasma cells. *Blood* 1999; 94(2):701-712.

[27] Archelos JJ, Storch MK, Hartung HP. The role of B cells and autoantibodies in multiple sclerosis. *Ann. Neurol.* 2000; 47(6):694-706.

[28] Cepok S, Jacobsen M, Schock S, Omer B, Jaekel S, Boddeker I, Oertel WH, Sommer N, Hemmer B. Patterns of cerebrospinal fluid pathology correlate with disease progression in multiple sclerosis. *Brain* 2001; 124(Pt 11):2169-2176.

[29] Cross AH, Trotter JL, Lyons J. B cells and antibodies in CNS demyelinating disease. *J. Neuroimmunol.* 2001; 112(1-2):1-14.

[30] Dalakas MC. B cells as therapeutic targets in autoimmune neurological disorders. *Nat. Clin. Pract. Neurol.* 2008; 4(10):557-567.

[31] Qin Y, Duquette P. B-cell immunity in MS. *Int MS J* 2003; 10(4):110-120.

[32] Bhakdi S, Tranum-Jensen J. Complement lysis: a hole is a hole. *Immunol. Today* 1991; 12(9):318-320.

[33] Duddy ME, Alter A, Bar-Or A. Distinct profiles of human B cell effector cytokines: a role in immune regulation? *J. Immunol.* 2004; 172(6):3422-3427.

[34] Ziemssen T, Ziemssen F. The role of the humoral immune system in multiple sclerosis (MS) and its animal model experimental autoimmune encephalomyelitis (EAE). *Autoimmun. Rev.* 2005; 4(7):460-467.

[35] Lanzavecchia A. Receptor-mediated antigen uptake and its effect on antigen presentation to class II-restricted T lymphocytes. *Annu. Rev. Immunol.* 1990; 8:773-793.

[36] Rock KL, Benacerraf B, Abbas AK. Antigen presentation by hapten-specific B lymphocytes. I. Role of surface immunoglobulin receptors. *J. Exp. Med.* 1984; 160(4):1102-1113.

[37] Genc K, Dona DL, Reder AT. Increased CD80(+) B cells in active multiple sclerosis and reversal by interferon beta-1b therapy. *J. Clin. Invest.* 1997; 99(11):2664-2671.

[38] Niino M, Hirotani M, Miyazaki Y, Sasaki H. Memory and naive B-cell subsets in patients with multiple sclerosis. *Neurosci. Lett.* 2009; 464(1):74-78.

[39] Torcia M, Bracci-Laudiero L, Lucibello M, Nencioni L, Labardi D, Rubartelli A, Cozzolino F, Aloe L, Garaci E. Nerve growth factor is an autocrine survival factor for memory B lymphocytes. *Cell* 1996; 85(3):345-356.

[40] Kerschensteiner M, Gallmeier E, Behrens L, Leal VV, Misgeld T, Klinkert WE, Kolbeck R, Hoppe E, Oropeza-Wekerle RL, Bartke I, Stadelmann C, Lassmann H, Wekerle H, Hohlfeld R. Activated human T cells, B cells, and monocytes produce brain-derived neurotrophic factor in vitro and in inflammatory brain lesions: a neuroprotective role of inflammation? *J. Exp. Med.* 1999; 189(5):865-870.

[41] Vargas-Leal V, Bruno R, Derfuss T, Krumbholz M, Hohlfeld R, Meinl E. Expression and function of glial cell line-derived neurotrophic factor family ligands and their receptors on human immune cells. *J. Immunol.* 2005; 175(4):2301-2308.

[42] Alter A, Duddy M, Hebert S, Biernacki K, Prat A, Antel JP, Yong VW, Nuttall RK, Pennington CJ, Edwards DR, Bar-Or A. Determinants of human B cell migration across brain endothelial cells. *J. Immunol.* 2003; 170(9):4497-4505.

[43] Krumbholz M, Theil D, Cepok S, Hemmer B, Kivisakk P, Ransohoff RM, Hofbauer M, Farina C, Derfuss T, Hartle C, Newcombe J, Hohlfeld R, Meinl E. Chemokines in multiple sclerosis: CXCL12 and CXCL13 up-regulation is differentially linked to CNS immune cell recruitment. *Brain* 2006; 129(Pt 1):200-211.

[44] Avery DT, Kalled SL, Ellyard JI, Ambrose C, Bixler SA, Thien M, Brink R, Mackay F, Hodgkin PD, Tangye SG. BAFF selectively enhances the survival of plasmablasts generated from human memory B cells. *J. Clin. Invest.* 2003; 112(2):286-297.

[45] Schneider P. The role of APRIL and BAFF in lymphocyte activation. *Curr. Opin. Immunol. 2*005; 17(3):282-289.

[46] Meinl E, Derfuss T, Krumbholz M, Probstel AK, Hohlfeld R. Humoral autoimmunity in multiple sclerosis. *J. Neurol. Sci.* 2010.

[47] Krumbholz M, Theil D, Derfuss T, Rosenwald A, Schrader F, Monoranu CM, Kalled SL, Hess DM, Serafini B, Aloisi F, Wekerle H, Hohlfeld R, Meinl E. BAFF is produced by astrocytes and up-regulated in multiple sclerosis lesions and primary central nervous system lymphoma. *J. Exp. Med.* 2005; 201(2):195-200.

[48] Thangarajh M, Gomes A, Masterman T, Hillert J, Hjelmstrom P. Expression of B-cell-activating factor of the TNF family (BAFF) and its receptors in multiple sclerosis. *J. Neuroimmunol.* 2004; 152(1-2):183-190.

[49] Thangarajh M, Masterman T, Rot U, Duvefelt K, Brynedal B, Karrenbauer VD, Hillert J. Increased levels of APRIL (a proliferation-

inducing ligand) mRNA in multiple sclerosis. *J. Neuroimmunol.* 2005; 167(1-2):210-214.

[50] Serafini B, Rosicarelli B, Franciotta D, Magliozzi R, Reynolds R, Cinque P, Andreoni L, Trivedi P, Salvetti M, Faggioni A, Aloisi F. Dysregulated Epstein-Barr virus infection in the multiple sclerosis brain. *J. Exp. Med.* 2007; 204(12):2899-2912.

[51] Daridon C, Youinou P, Pers JO. BAFF, APRIL, TWE-PRIL: who's who? *Autoimmun. Rev.* 2008; 7(4):267-271.

[52] Laterre EC, Callewaert A, Heremans JF, Sfaello Z. Electrophoretic morphology of gamma globulins in cerebrospinal fluid of multiple sclerosis and other diseases of the nervous system. *Neurology* 1970; 20(10):982-990.

[53] Kabat EA, Glusman M, Knaub V. Quantitative estimation of the albumin and gamma-globulin in normal and pathological cerebrospinal fluid by immunochemical methods. *Am. J. Med.* 1948; 4:653-662.

[54] Irani D. Cerebrospinal fluid. In *Clinical Practice.* Philadelphia, USA: Saunders Elsevier, 2009.

[55] Walsh MJ, Tourtellotte WW. Temporal invariance and clonal uniformity of brain and cerebrospinal IgG, IgA, and IgM in multiple sclerosis. *J. Exp. Med.* 1986; 163(1):41-53.

[56] Walsh MJ, Tourtellotte WW. Temporal invariance and clonal uniformity of brain and cerebrospinal IgG, IgA, and IgM in multiple sclerosis. *J. Exp. Med.* 1986; 163(1):41-53.

[57] Freedman MS, Thompson EJ, Deisenhammer F, Giovannoni G, Grimsley G, Keir G, Ohman S, Racke MK, Sharief M, Sindic CJ, Sellebjerg F, Tourtellotte WW. Recommended standard of cerebrospinal fluid analysis in the diagnosis of multiple sclerosis: a consensus statement. *Arch. Neurol.* 2005; 62(6):865-870.

[58] McDonald WI, Compston A, Edan G, Goodkin D, Hartung HP, Lublin FD, McFarland HF, Paty DW, Polman CH, Reingold SC, Sandberg-Wollheim M, Sibley W, Thompson A, Van Den NS, Weinshenker BY, Wolinsky JS. Recommended diagnostic criteria for multiple sclerosis: guidelines from the International Panel on the diagnosis of multiple sclerosis. *Ann. Neurol.* 2001; 50(1):121-127.

[59] Qin Y, Duquette P, Zhang Y, Olek M, Da RR, Richardson J, Antel JP, Talbot P, Cashman NR, Tourtellotte WW, Wekerle H, Van Den NS. Intrathecal B-cell clonal expansion, an early sign of humoral immunity, in the cerebrospinal fluid of patients with clinically isolated syndrome suggestive of multiple sclerosis. *Lab. Invest.* 2003; 83(7):1081-1088.

[60] Baranzini SE, Jeong MC, Butunoi C, Murray RS, Bernard CC, Oksenberg JR. B cell repertoire diversity and clonal expansion in multiple sclerosis brain lesions. *J. Immunol.* 1999; 163(9):5133-5144.

[61] Cepok S, Rosche B, Grummel V, Vogel F, Zhou D, Sayn J, Sommer N, Hartung HP, Hemmer B. Short-lived plasma blasts are the main B cell effector subset during the course of multiple sclerosis. *Brain* 2005; 128(Pt 7):1667-1676.

[62] Genain CP, Cannella B, Hauser SL, Raine CS. Identification of autoantibodies associated with myelin damage in multiple sclerosis. *Nat. Med.* 1999; 5(2):170-175.

[63] Lassmann H, Bruck W, Lucchinetti C. Heterogeneity of multiple sclerosis pathogenesis: implications for diagnosis and therapy. *Trends. Mol. Med.* 2001; 7(3):115-121.

[64] Cross AH, Trotter JL, Lyons J. B cells and antibodies in CNS demyelinating disease. *J. Neuroimmunol.* 2001; 112(1-2):1-14.

[65] Lucchinetti C, Bruck W, Parisi J, Scheithauer B, Rodriguez M, Lassmann H. Heterogeneity of multiple sclerosis lesions: implications for the pathogenesis of demyelination. *Ann. Neurol.* 2000; 47(6):707-717.

[66] Serafini B, Rosicarelli B, Magliozzi R, Stigliano E, Aloisi F. Detection of ectopic B-cell follicles with germinal centers in the meninges of patients with secondary progressive multiple sclerosis. *Brain. Pathol.* 2004; 14(2):164-174.

[67] Corcione A, Aloisi F, Serafini B, Capello E, Mancardi GL, Pistoia V, Uccelli A. B-cell differentiation in the CNS of patients with multiple sclerosis. *Autoimmun. Rev.* 2005; 4(8):549-554.

[68] Aloisi F, Serafini B, Magliozzi R, Howell OW, Reynolds R. *Detection of Epstein-Barr virus and B-cell follicles in the multiple sclerosis brain: what you find depends on how and where you look.* Brain 2010.

[69] Magliozzi R, Columba-Cabezas S, Serafini B, Aloisi F. Intracerebral expression of CXCL13 and BAFF is accompanied by formation of lymphoid follicle-like structures in the meninges of mice with relapsing experimental autoimmune encephalomyelitis. *J. Neuroimmunol.* 2004; 148(1-2):11-23.

[70] Izquierdo G, Angulo S, Garcia-Moreno JM, Gamero MA, Navarro G, Gata JM, Ruiz-Pena JL, Paramo MD. Intrathecal IgG synthesis: marker of progression in multiple sclerosis patients. *Acta Neurol. Scand.* 2002; 105(3):158-163.

[71] Linington C, Bradl M, Lassmann H, Brunner C, Vass K. Augmentation of demyelination in rat acute allergic encephalomyelitis by circulating mouse monoclonal antibodies directed against a myelin/oligodendrocyte glycoprotein. *Am. J. Pathol.* 1988; 130(3):443-454.

[72] Morris-Downes MM, Smith PA, Rundle JL, Piddlesden SJ, Baker D, Pham-Dinh D, Heijmans N, Amor S. Pathological and regulatory effects of anti-myelin antibodies in experimental allergic encephalomyelitis in mice. *J. Neuroimmunol.* 2002; 125(1-2):114-124.

[73] Mathey EK, Derfuss T, Storch MK, Williams KR, Hales K, Woolley DR, Al Hayani A, Davies SN, Rasband MN, Olsson T, Moldenhauer A, Velhin S, Hohlfeld R, Meinl E, Linington C. Neurofascin as a novel target for autoantibody-mediated axonal injury. *J. Exp. Med.* 2007; 204(10):2363-2372.

[74] Martin MP, Monson NL. Potential role of humoral immunity in the pathogenesis of multiple sclerosis (MS) and experimental autoimmune encephalomyelitis (EAE). *Front Biosci.* 2007; 12:2735-2749.

[75] Keegan M, Konig F, McClelland R, Bruck W, Morales Y, Bitsch A, Panitch H, Lassmann H, Weinshenker B, Rodriguez M, Parisi J, Lucchinetti CF. Relation between humoral pathological changes in multiple sclerosis and response to therapeutic plasma exchange. *Lancet* 2005; 366(9485):579-582.

[76] Cross AH, Stark JL, Lauber J, Ramsbottom MJ, Lyons JA. Rituximab reduces B cells and T cells in cerebrospinal fluid of multiple sclerosis patients. *J. Neuroimmunol.* 2006; 180(1-2):63-70.

[77] Hauser SL, Waubant E, Arnold DL, Vollmer T, Antel J, Fox RJ, Bar-Or A, Panzara M, Sarkar N, Agarwal S, Langer-Gould A, Smith CH. B-cell depletion with rituximab in relapsing-remitting multiple sclerosis. *N. Engl. J. Med.* 2008; 358(7):676-688.

[78] Kerschensteiner M, Gallmeier E, Behrens L, Leal VV, Misgeld T, Klinkert WE, Kolbeck R, Hoppe E, Oropeza-Wekerle RL, Bartke I, Stadelmann C, Lassmann H, Wekerle H, Hohlfeld R. Activated human T cells, B cells, and monocytes produce brain-derived neurotrophic factor in vitro and in inflammatory brain lesions: a neuroprotective role of inflammation? *J. Exp. Med.* 1999; 189(5):865-870.

[79] Fillatreau S, Sweenie CH, McGeachy MJ, Gray D, Anderton SM. B cells regulate autoimmunity by provision of IL-10. *Nat. Immunol.* 2002; 3(10):944-950.

[80] Warrington AE, Asakura K, Bieber AJ, Ciric B, Van K, V, Kaveri SV, Kyle RA, Pease LR, Rodriguez M. Human monoclonal antibodies

reactive to oligodendrocytes promote remyelination in a model of multiple sclerosis. *Proc. Natl. Acad. Sci. USA* 2000; 97(12):6820-6825.

[81] Cross AH, Trotter JL, Lyons J. B cells and antibodies in CNS demyelinating disease. *J. Neuroimmunol.* 2001; 112(1-2):1-14.

[82] Cepok S, Zhou D, Srivastava R, Nessler S, Stei S, Bussow K, Sommer N, Hemmer B. Identification of Epstein-Barr virus proteins as putative targets of the immune response in multiple sclerosis. *J. Clin. Invest.* 2005; 115(5):1352-1360.

[83] Quintana FJ, Farez MF, Viglietta V, Iglesias AH, Merbl Y, Izquierdo G, Lucas M, Basso AS, Khoury SJ, Lucchinetti CF, Cohen IR, Weiner HL. Antigen microarrays identify unique serum autoantibody signatures in clinical and pathologic subtypes of multiple sclerosis. *Proc. Natl. Acad. Sci. USA* 2008; 105(48):18889-18894.

[84] Zhou D, Srivastava R, Nessler S, Grummel V, Sommer N, Bruck W, Hartung HP, Stadelmann C, Hemmer B. Identification of a pathogenic antibody response to native myelin oligodendrocyte glycoprotein in multiple sclerosis. *Proc. Natl. Acad. Sci. USA* 2006; 103(50):19057-19062.

[85] Reindl M, Khalil M, Berger T. Antibodies as biological markers for pathophysiological processes in MS. *J. Neuroimmunol.* 2006; 180(1-2):50-62.

[86] Huizinga R, Linington C, Amor S. Resistance is futile: antineuronal autoimmunity in multiple sclerosis. *Trends Immunol.* 2008; 29(2):54-60.

[87] Reindl M, Linington C, Brehm U, Egg R, Dilitz E, Deisenhammer F, Poewe W, Berger T. Antibodies against the myelin oligodendrocyte glycoprotein and the myelin basic protein in multiple sclerosis and other neurological diseases: a comparative study. *Brain* 1999; 122 (Pt 11):2047-2056.

[88] Reindl M, Linington C, Brehm U, Egg R, Dilitz E, Deisenhammer F, Poewe W, Berger T. Antibodies against the myelin oligodendrocyte glycoprotein and the myelin basic protein in multiple sclerosis and other neurological diseases: a comparative study. *Brain* 1999; 122 (Pt 11):2047-2056.

[89] Sun JB, Olsson T, Wang WZ, Xiao BG, Kostulas V, Fredrikson S, Ekre HP, Link H. Autoreactive T and B cells responding to myelin proteolipid protein in multiple sclerosis and controls. *Eur. J. Immunol.* 1991; 21(6):1461-1468.

[90] Moller JR, Johnson D, Brady RO, Tourtellotte WW, Quarles RH. Antibodies to myelin-associated glycoprotein (MAG) in the

cerebrospinal fluid of multiple sclerosis patients. *J. Neuroimmunol.* 1989; 22(1):55-61.

[91] O'Connor KC, Chitnis T, Griffin DE, Piyasirisilp S, Bar-Or A, Khoury S, Wucherpfennig KW, Hafler DA. Myelin basic protein-reactive autoantibodies in the serum and cerebrospinal fluid of multiple sclerosis patients are characterized by low-affinity interactions. *J. Neuroimmunol.* 2003; 136(1-2):140-148.

[92] Pittock SJ, Reindl M, Achenbach S, Berger T, Bruck W, Konig F, Morales Y, Lassmann H, Bryant S, Moore SB, Keegan BM, Lucchinetti CF. Myelin oligodendrocyte glycoprotein antibodies in pathologically proven multiple sclerosis: frequency, stability and clinicopathologic correlations. *Mult. Scler.* 2007; 13(1):7-16.

[93] Lim ET, Berger T, Reindl M, Dalton CM, Fernando K, Keir G, Thompson EJ, Miller DH, Giovannoni G. Anti-myelin antibodies do not allow earlier diagnosis of multiple sclerosis. *Mult. Scler.* 2005; 11(4):492-494.

[94] Reindl M, Linington C, Brehm U, Egg R, Dilitz E, Deisenhammer F, Poewe W, Berger T. Antibodies against the myelin oligodendrocyte glycoprotein and the myelin basic protein in multiple sclerosis and other neurological diseases: a comparative study. *Brain* 1999; 122 (Pt 11):2047-2056.

[95] Reindl M, Khalil M, Berger T. Antibodies as biological markers for pathophysiological processes in MS. *J. Neuroimmunol.* 2006; 180(1-2):50-62.

[96] Huizinga R, Linington C, Amor S. Resistance is futile: antineuronal autoimmunity in multiple sclerosis. *Trends Immunol.* 2008; 29(2):54-60.

[97] Agius MA, Kirvan CA, Schafer AL, Gudipati E, Zhu S. High prevalence of anti-alpha-crystallin antibodies in multiple sclerosis: correlation with severity and activity of disease. *Acta. Neurol. Scand.* 1999; 100(3):139-147.

[98] Williamson RA, Burgoon MP, Owens GP, Ghausi O, Leclerc E, Firme L, Carlson S, Corboy J, Parren PW, Sanna PP, Gilden DH, Burton DR. Anti-DNA antibodies are a major component of the intrathecal B cell response in multiple sclerosis. *Proc. Natl. Acad. Sci. USA* 2001; 98(4):1793-1798.

[99] Tozzoli R. Recent advances in diagnostic technologies and their impact in autoimmune diseases. *Autoimmun. Rev.* 2007; 6(6):334-340.

[100] Plebani M, Pittoni M, Celadin M, Bernardi D, Mion MM. Recent advances in diagnostic technologies for autoimmune diseases. *Autoimmun. Rev.* 2009; 8(3):238-243.

[101] Blass S, Engel JM, Burmester GR. The immunologic homunculus in rheumatoid arthritis. *Arthritis Rheum.* 1999; 42(12):2499-2506.

[102] Stinton LM, Fritzler MJ. A clinical approach to autoantibody testing in systemic autoimmune rheumatic disorders. *Autoimmun. Rev.* 2007; 7(1):77-84.

[103] Kanter JL, Narayana S, Ho PP, Catz I, Warren KG, Sobel RA, Steinman L, Robinson WH. Lipid microarrays identify key mediators of autoimmune brain inflammation. *Nat. Med.* 2006; 12(1):138-143.

[104] Quintana FJ, Farez MF, Viglietta V, Iglesias AH, Merbl Y, Izquierdo G, Lucas M, Basso AS, Khoury SJ, Lucchinetti CF, Cohen IR, Weiner HL. Antigen microarrays identify unique serum autoantibody signatures in clinical and pathologic subtypes of multiple sclerosis. *Proc. Natl. Acad. Sci. USA* 2008; 105(48):18889-18894.

[105] Quintana FJ, Farez MF, Viglietta V, Iglesias AH, Merbl Y, Izquierdo G, Lucas M, Basso AS, Khoury SJ, Lucchinetti CF, Cohen IR, Weiner HL. Antigen microarrays identify unique serum autoantibody signatures in clinical and pathologic subtypes of multiple sclerosis. *Proc. Natl. Acad. Sci. USA* 2008; 105(48):18889-18894.

[106] Cepok S, Zhou D, Srivastava R, Nessler S, Stei S, Bussow K, Sommer N, Hemmer B. Identification of Epstein-Barr virus proteins as putative targets of the immune response in multiple sclerosis. *J. Clin. Invest.* 2005; 115(5):1352-1360.

[107] Cepok S, Zhou D, Srivastava R, Nessler S, Stei S, Bussow K, Sommer N, Hemmer B. Identification of Epstein-Barr virus proteins as putative targets of the immune response in multiple sclerosis. *J. Clin. Invest.* 2005; 115(5):1352-1360.

[108] Lefranc D, Almeras L, Dubucquoi S, de Seze J, Vermersch P, Prin L. Distortion of the self-reactive IgG antibody repertoire in multiple sclerosis as a new diagnostic tool. *J. Immunol.* 2004; 172(1):669-678.

[109] Lefranc D, Almeras L, Dubucquoi S, de Seze J, Vermersch P, Prin L. Distortion of the self-reactive IgG antibody repertoire in multiple sclerosis as a new diagnostic tool. *J. Immunol.* 2004; 172(1):669-678.

[110] Kolln J, Ren HM, Da RR, Zhang Y, Spillner E, Olek M, Hermanowicz N, Hilgenberg LG, Smith MA, Van Den NS, Qin Y. Triosephosphate isomerase- and glyceraldehyde-3-phosphate dehydrogenase-reactive

autoantibodies in the cerebrospinal fluid of patients with multiple sclerosis. *J. Immunol.* 2006; 177(8):5652-5658.

[111] Mathey EK, Derfuss T, Storch MK, Williams KR, Hales K, Woolley DR, Al Hayani A, Davies SN, Rasband MN, Olsson T, Moldenhauer A, Velhin S, Hohlfeld R, Meinl E, Linington C. Neurofascin as a novel target for autoantibody-mediated axonal injury. *J. Exp. Med.* 2007; 204(10):2363-2372.

[112] Derfuss T, Parikh K, Velhin S, Braun M, Mathey E, Krumbholz M, Kumpfel T, Moldenhauer A, Rader C, Sonderegger P, Pollmann W, Tiefenthaller C, Bauer J, Lassmann H, Wekerle H, Karagogeos D, Hohlfeld R, Linington C, Meinl E. Contactin-2/TAG-1-directed autoimmunity is identified in multiple sclerosis patients and mediates gray matter pathology in animals. *Proc. Natl. Acad. Sci. USA* 2009.

[113] Mathey EK, Derfuss T, Storch MK, Williams KR, Hales K, Woolley DR, Al Hayani A, Davies SN, Rasband MN, Olsson T, Moldenhauer A, Velhin S, Hohlfeld R, Meinl E, Linington C. Neurofascin as a novel target for autoantibody-mediated axonal injury. *J. Exp. Med.* 2007; 204(10):2363-2372.

[114] Derfuss T, Parikh K, Velhin S, Braun M, Mathey E, Krumbholz M, Kumpfel T, Moldenhauer A, Rader C, Sonderegger P, Pollmann W, Tiefenthaller C, Bauer J, Lassmann H, Wekerle H, Karagogeos D, Hohlfeld R, Linington C, Meinl E. Contactin-2/TAG-1-directed autoimmunity is identified in multiple sclerosis patients and mediates gray matter pathology in animals. *Proc. Natl. Acad. Sci. USA* 2009.

[115] Reindl M, Linington C, Brehm U, Egg R, Dilitz E, Deisenhammer F, Poewe W, Berger T. Antibodies against the myelin oligodendrocyte glycoprotein and the myelin basic protein in multiple sclerosis and other neurological diseases: a comparative study. *Brain* 1999; 122 (Pt 11):2047-2056.

[116] Olsson T, Baig S, Hojeberg B, Link H. Antimyelin basic protein and antimyelin antibody-producing cells in multiple sclerosis. *Ann. Neurol.* 1990; 27(2):132-136.

[117] Reindl M, Linington C, Brehm U, Egg R, Dilitz E, Deisenhammer F, Poewe W, Berger T. Antibodies against the myelin oligodendrocyte glycoprotein and the myelin basic protein in multiple sclerosis and other neurological diseases: a comparative study. *Brain* 1999; 122 (Pt 11):2047-2056.

[118] Moller JR, Johnson D, Brady RO, Tourtellotte WW, Quarles RH. Antibodies to myelin-associated glycoprotein (MAG) in the

cerebrospinal fluid of multiple sclerosis patients. *J. Neuroimmunol.* 1989; 22(1):55-61.

[119] Sun JB, Olsson T, Wang WZ, Xiao BG, Kostulas V, Fredrikson S, Ekre HP, Link H. Autoreactive T and B cells responding to myelin proteolipid protein in multiple sclerosis and controls. *Eur. J. Immunol.* 1991; 21(6):1461-1468.

[120] Lolli F, Mazzanti B, Pazzagli M, Peroni E, Alcaro MC, Sabatino G, Lanzillo R, Brescia M, V, Santoro L, Gasperini C, Galgani S, D'Elios MM, Zipoli V, Sotgiu S, Pugliatti M, Rovero P, Chelli M, Papini AM. The glycopeptide CSF114(Glc) detects serum antibodies in multiple sclerosis. *J. Neuroimmunol.* 2005; 167(1-2):131-137.

[121] Schwarz M, Spector L, Gortler M, Weisshaus O, Glass-Marmor L, Karni A, Dotan N, Miller A. Serum anti-Glc(alpha1,4)Glc(alpha) antibodies as a biomarker for relapsing-remitting multiple sclerosis. *J. Neurol. Sci.* 2006; 244(1-2):59-68.

[122] Villar LM, Sadaba MC, Roldan E, Masjuan J, Gonzalez-Porque P, Villarrubia N, Espino M, Garcia-Trujillo JA, Bootello A, Alvarez-Cermeno JC. Intrathecal synthesis of oligoclonal IgM against myelin lipids predicts an aggressive disease course in MS. *J. Clin. Invest.* 2005; 115(1):187-194.

[123] Kanter JL, Narayana S, Ho PP, Catz I, Warren KG, Sobel RA, Steinman L, Robinson WH. Lipid microarrays identify key mediators of autoimmune brain inflammation. *Nat. Med.* 2006; 12(1):138-143.

[124] Menge T, Lalive PH, von Budingen HC, Cree B, Hauser SL, Genain CP. Antibody responses against galactocerebroside are potential stage-specific biomarkers in multiple sclerosis. *J. Allergy Clin. Immunol.* 2005; 116(2):453-459.

[125] Zanetta JP, Tranchant C, Kuchler-Bopp S, Lehmann S, Warter JM. Presence of anti-CSL antibodies in the cerebrospinal fluid of patients: a sensitive and specific test in the diagnosis of multiple sclerosis. *J. Neuroimmunol.* 1994; 52(2):175-182.

[126] Silber E, Semra YK, Gregson NA, Sharief MK. Patients with progressive multiple sclerosis have elevated antibodies to neurofilament subunit. *Neurology* 2002; 58(9):1372-1381.

[127] Sadatipour BT, Greer JM, Pender MP. Increased circulating antiganglioside antibodies in primary and secondary progressive multiple sclerosis. *Ann. Neurol.* 1998; 44(6):980-983.

[128] Rawes JA, Calabrese VP, Khan OA, DeVries GH. Antibodies to the axolemma-enriched fraction in the cerebrospinal fluid and serum of

patients with multiple sclerosis and other neurological diseases. *Mult. Scler.* 1997; 3(6):363-369.

[129] Svarcova J, Fialova L, Bartos A, Steinbachova M, Malbohan I. Cerebrospinal fluid antibodies to tubulin are elevated in the patients with multiple sclerosis. *Eur. J. Neurol.* 2008; 15(11):1173-1179.

[130] Reindl M, Khantane S, Ehling R, Schanda K, Lutterotti A, Brinkhoff C, Oertle T, Schwab ME, Deisenhammer F, Berger T, Bandtlow CE. Serum and cerebrospinal fluid antibodies to Nogo-A in patients with multiple sclerosis and acute neurological disorders. *J. Neuroimmunol.* 2003; 145(1-2):139-147.

[131] Onoue H, Satoh JI, Ogawa M, Tabunoki H, Yamamura T. Detection of anti-Nogo receptor autoantibody in the serum of multiple sclerosis and controls. *Acta Neurol. Scand.* 2007; 115(3):153-160.

[132] Lily O, Palace J, Vincent A. Serum autoantibodies to cell surface determinants in multiple sclerosis: a flow cytometric study. *Brain* 2004; 127(Pt 2):269-279.

[133] Mathey EK, Derfuss T, Storch MK, Williams KR, Hales K, Woolley DR, Al Hayani A, Davies SN, Rasband MN, Olsson T, Moldenhauer A, Velhin S, Hohlfeld R, Meinl E, Linington C. Neurofascin as a novel target for autoantibody-mediated axonal injury. *J. Exp. Med.* 2007; 204(10):2363-2372.

[134] Derfuss T, Parikh K, Velhin S, Braun M, Mathey E, Krumbholz M, Kumpfel T, Moldenhauer A, Rader C, Sonderegger P, Pollmann W, Tiefenthaller C, Bauer J, Lassmann H, Wekerle H, Karagogeos D, Hohlfeld R, Linington C, Meinl E. Contactin-2/TAG-1-directed autoimmunity is identified in multiple sclerosis patients and mediates gray matter pathology in animals. *Proc. Natl. Acad. Sci. USA* 2009.

[135] Lily O, Palace J, Vincent A. Serum autoantibodies to cell surface determinants in multiple sclerosis: a flow cytometric study. *Brain* 2004; 127(Pt 2):269-279.

[136] Niehaus A, Shi J, Grzenkowski M, Diers-Fenger M, Archelos J, Hartung HP, Toyka K, Bruck W, Trotter J. Patients with active relapsing-remitting multiple sclerosis synthesize antibodies recognizing oligodendrocyte progenitor cell surface protein: implications for remyelination. *Ann. Neurol.* 2000; 48(3):362-371.

[137] Bronstein JM, Lallone RL, Seitz RS, Ellison GW, Myers LW. A humoral response to oligodendrocyte-specific protein in MS: a potential molecular mimic. *Neurology* 1999; 53(1):154-161.

[138] Banki K, Colombo E, Sia F, Halladay D, Mattson DH, Tatum AH, Massa PT, Phillips PE, Perl A. Oligodendrocyte-specific expression and autoantigenicity of transaldolase in multiple sclerosis. *J. Exp. Med.* 1994; 180(5):1649-1663.

[139] Walsh MJ, Murray JM. Dual implication of 2',3'-cyclic nucleotide 3' phosphodiesterase as major autoantigen and C3 complement-binding protein in the pathogenesis of multiple sclerosis. *J. Clin. Invest.* 1998; 101(9):1923-1931.

[140] Agius MA, Kirvan CA, Schafer AL, Gudipati E, Zhu S. High prevalence of anti-alpha-crystallin antibodies in multiple sclerosis: correlation with severity and activity of disease. *Acta. Neurol. Scand.* 1999; 100(3):139-147.

[141] Selmaj K, Brosnan CF, Raine CS. Expression of heat shock protein-65 by oligodendrocytes in vivo and in vitro: implications for multiple sclerosis. *Neurology* 1992; 42(4):795-800.

[142] Chiba S, Yokota S, Yonekura K, Tanaka S, Furuyama H, Kubota H, Fujii N, Matsumoto H. Autoantibodies against HSP70 family proteins were detected in the cerebrospinal fluid from patients with multiple sclerosis. *J. Neurol. Sci.* 2006; 241(1-2):39-43.

[143] Cid C, Alvarez-Cermeno JC, Salinas M, Alcazar A. Anti-heat shock protein 90beta antibodies decrease pre-oligodendrocyte population in perinatal and adult cell cultures. Implications for remyelination in multiple sclerosis. *J. Neurochem.* 2005; 95(2):349-360.

[144] Mayo I, Arribas J, Villoslada P, Alvarez DR, Rodriguez-Vilarino S, Montalban X, De Sagarra MR, Castano JG. The proteasome is a major autoantigen in multiple sclerosis. *Brain* 2002; 125(Pt 12):2658-2667.

[145] Williamson RA, Burgoon MP, Owens GP, Ghausi O, Leclerc E, Firme L, Carlson S, Corboy J, Parren PW, Sanna PP, Gilden DH, Burton DR. Anti-DNA antibodies are a major component of the intrathecal B cell response in multiple sclerosis. *Proc. Natl. Acad. Sci. USA* 2001; 98(4):1793-1798.

[146] Sueoka E, Yukitake M, Iwanaga K, Sueoka N, Aihara T, Kuroda Y. Autoantibodies against heterogeneous nuclear ribonucleoprotein B1 in CSF of MS patients. *Ann. Neurol.* 2004; 56(6):778-786.

[147] Gorczyca WA, Ejma M, Witkowska D, Misiuk-Hojlo M, Kuropatwa M, Mulak M, Szymaniec S. Retinal antigens are recognized by antibodies present in sera of patients with multiple sclerosis. *Ophthalmic. Res.* 2004; 36(2):120-123.

[148] Kolln J, Ren HM, Da RR, Zhang Y, Spillner E, Olek M, Hermanowicz N, Hilgenberg LG, Smith MA, Van Den NS, Qin Y. Triosephosphate isomerase- and glyceraldehyde-3-phosphate dehydrogenase-reactive autoantibodies in the cerebrospinal fluid of patients with multiple sclerosis. *J. Immunol.* 2006; 177(8):5652-5658.

[149] Kolln J, Ren HM, Da RR, Zhang Y, Spillner E, Olek M, Hermanowicz N, Hilgenberg LG, Smith MA, Van Den NS, Qin Y. Triosephosphate isomerase- and glyceraldehyde-3-phosphate dehydrogenase-reactive autoantibodies in the cerebrospinal fluid of patients with multiple sclerosis. *J. Immunol.* 2006; 177(8):5652-5658.

[150] Archelos JJ, Trotter J, Previtali S, Weissbrich B, Toyka KV, Hartung HP. Isolation and characterization of an oligodendrocyte precursor-derived B-cell epitope in multiple sclerosis. *Ann. Neurol.* 1998; 43(1):15-24.

[151] Cepok S, Zhou D, Srivastava R, Nessler S, Stei S, Bussow K, Sommer N, Hemmer B. Identification of Epstein-Barr virus proteins as putative targets of the immune response in multiple sclerosis. *J. Clin. Invest.* 2005; 115(5):1352-1360.

[152] Cepok S, Zhou D, Srivastava R, Nessler S, Stei S, Bussow K, Sommer N, Hemmer B. Identification of Epstein-Barr virus proteins as putative targets of the immune response in multiple sclerosis. *J. Clin. Invest.* 2005; 115(5):1352-1360.

[153] Reindl M, Khalil M, Berger T. Antibodies as biological markers for pathophysiological processes in MS. *J. Neuroimmunol.* 2006; 180(1-2):50-62.

[154] Huizinga R, Linington C, Amor S. Resistance is futile: antineuronal autoimmunity in multiple sclerosis. *Trends Immunol.* 2008; 29(2):54-60.

[155] Archelos JJ, Trotter J, Previtali S, Weissbrich B, Toyka KV, Hartung HP. Isolation and characterization of an oligodendrocyte precursor-derived B-cell epitope in multiple sclerosis. *Ann. Neurol.* 1998; 43(1):15-24.

[156] Archelos JJ, Trotter J, Previtali S, Weissbrich B, Toyka KV, Hartung HP. Isolation and characterization of an oligodendrocyte precursor-derived B-cell epitope in multiple sclerosis. *Ann. Neurol.* 1998; 43(1):15-24.

[157] Owens GP, Burgoon MP, Devlin ME, Gilden DH. Strategies to identify sequences or antigens unique to multiple sclerosis. *Mult. Scler.* 1996; 2(4):184-194.

[158] Smith GP. Filamentous fusion phage: novel expression vectors that display cloned antigens on the virion surface. *Science* 1985; 228(4705):1315-1317.

[159] Smith GP. Filamentous fusion phage: novel expression vectors that display cloned antigens on the virion surface. *Science* 1985; 228(4705):1315-1317.

[160] Webster R. Biology of the Filamentous Bacteriophage. In: Kay B, Winter J, McCafferty J, editors. *Phage Display of Peptides and Proteins. A laboratory Manual.* San Diego, California: Academic Press, INC, 1996: 1-20.

[161] Smith GP. Filamentous fusion phage: novel expression vectors that display cloned antigens on the virion surface. *Science* 1985; 228(4705):1315-1317.

[162] Archelos JJ, Trotter J, Previtali S, Weissbrich B, Toyka KV, Hartung HP. Isolation and characterization of an oligodendrocyte precursor-derived B-cell epitope in multiple sclerosis. *Ann. Neurol.* 1998; 43(1):15-24.

[163] Owens GP, Burgoon MP, Devlin ME, Gilden DH. Strategies to identify sequences or antigens unique to multiple sclerosis. *Mult. Scler.* 1996; 2(4):184-194.

[164] Scott JK, Smith GP. Searching for peptide ligands with an epitope library. *Science* 1990; 249(4967):386-390.

[165] Cortese I, Tafi R, Grimaldi LM, Martino G, Nicosia A, Cortese R. Identification of peptides specific for cerebrospinal fluid antibodies in multiple sclerosis by using phage libraries. *Proc. Natl. Acad. Sci. USA* 1996; 93(20):11063-11067.

[166] Cortese I, Capone S, Luchetti S, Grimaldi LM, Nicosia A, Cortese R. CSF-enriched antibodies do not share specificities among MS patients. *Mult. Scler.* 1998; 4(3):118-123.

[167] Dybwad A, Flrre O, Sioud M. Probing for cerebrospinal fluid antibody specificities by a panel of random peptide libraries. *Autoimmunity* 1997; 25(2):85-89.

[168] Jolivet-Reynaud C, Perron H, Ferrante P, Becquart L, Dalbon P, Mandrand B. Specificities of multiple sclerosis cerebrospinal fluid and serum antibodies against mimotopes. *Clin. Immunol.* 1999; 93(3):283-293.

[169] Rand KH, Houck H, Denslow ND, Heilman KM. Molecular approach to find target(s) for oligoclonal bands in multiple sclerosis. *J. Neurol. Neurosurg. Psychiatry* 1998; 65(1):48-55.

[170] Rand KH, Houck H, Denslow ND, Heilman KM. Epstein-Barr virus nuclear antigen-1 (EBNA-1) associated oligoclonal bands in patients with multiple sclerosis. *J. Neurol. Sci.* 2000; 173(1):32-39.

[171] Cortese I, Capone S, Luchetti S, Cortese R, Nicosia A. Cross-reactive phage-displayed mimotopes lead to the discovery of mimicry between HSV-1 and a brain-specific protein. *J. Neuroimmunol.* 2001; 113(1):119-128.

[172] Cortese I, Capone S, Luchetti S, Cortese R, Nicosia A. Cross-reactive phage-displayed mimotopes lead to the discovery of mimicry between HSV-1 and a brain-specific protein. *J. Neuroimmunol.* 2001; 113(1):119-128.

[173] Hufton SE, Moerkerk PT, Meulemans EV, de Bruine A, Arends JW, Hoogenboom HR. Phage display of cDNA repertoires: the pVI display system and its applications for the selection of immunogenic ligands. *J. Immunol. Methods* 1999; 231(1-2):39-51.

[174] Becker KG, Mattson DH, Powers JM, Gado AM, Biddison WE. Analysis of a sequenced cDNA library from multiple sclerosis lesions. *J. Neuroimmunol.* 1997; 77(1):27-38.

[175] Becker KG, Mattson DH, Powers JM, Gado AM, Biddison WE. Analysis of a sequenced cDNA library from multiple sclerosis lesions. *J. Neuroimmunol.* 1997; 77(1):27-38.

[176] Becker KG, Mattson DH, Powers JM, Gado AM, Biddison WE. Analysis of a sequenced cDNA library from multiple sclerosis lesions. *J. Neuroimmunol.* 1997; 77(1):27-38.

[177] Somers V, Govarts C, Somers K, Hupperts R, Medaer R, Stinissen P. Autoantibody profiling in multiple sclerosis reveals novel antigenic candidates. *J. Immunol.* 2008; 180(6):3957-3963.

[178] Somers V, Govarts C, Somers K, Hupperts R, Medaer R, Stinissen P. Autoantibody profiling in multiple sclerosis reveals novel antigenic candidates. *J. Immunol.* 2008; 180(6):3957-3963.

[179] Link H, Baig S, Jiang YP, Olsson O, Hojeberg B, Kostulas V, Olsson T. B cells and antibodies in MS. *Res. Immunol.* 1989; 140(2):219-226.

[180] Sun J, Link H, Olsson T, Xiao BG, Andersson G, Ekre HP, Linington C, Diener P. T and B cell responses to myelin-oligodendrocyte glycoprotein in multiple sclerosis. *J. Immunol.* 1991; 146(5):1490-1495.

[181] Lambracht-Washington D, O'connor KC, Cameron EM, Jowdry A, Ward ES, Frohman E, Racke MK, Monson NL. Antigen specificity of clonally expanded and receptor edited cerebrospinal fluid B cells from patients with relapsing remitting MS. *J. Neuroimmunol.* 2007.

[182] von Budingen HC, Harrer MD, Kuenzle S, Meier M, Goebels N. Clonally expanded plasma cells in the cerebrospinal fluid of MS patients produce myelin-specific antibodies. *Eur. J. Immunol.* 2008; 38(7):2014-2023.

[183] Zhang Y, Da RR, Guo W, Ren HM, Hilgenberg LG, Sobel RA, Tourtellotte WW, Smith MA, Olek M, Gupta S, Robertson RT, Nagra R, van den NS, Qin Y. Axon reactive B cells clonally expanded in the cerebrospinal fluid of patients with multiple sclerosis. *J. Clin. Immunol.* 2005; 25(3):254-264.

[184] Kolln J, Ren HM, Da RR, Zhang Y, Spillner E, Olek M, Hermanowicz N, Hilgenberg LG, Smith MA, van den NS, Qin Y. Triosephosphate isomerase- and glyceraldehyde-3-phosphate dehydrogenase-reactive autoantibodies in the cerebrospinal fluid of patients with multiple sclerosis. *J. Immunol.* 2006; 177(8):5652-5658.

[185] Yu X, Gilden D, Schambers L, Barmina O, Burgoon M, Bennett J, Owens G. Peptide reactivity between multiple sclerosis (MS) CSF IgG and recombinant antibodies generated from clonally expanded plasma cells in MS CSF. *J. Neuroimmunol.* 2010.

[186] Martin DR, Marlowe RL, Ahearn JM. Determination of the role for CD21 during Epstein-Barr virus infection of B-lymphoblastoid cells. *J. Virol.* 1994; 68(8):4716-4726.

[187] Sugimoto M, Tahara H, Ide T, Furuichi Y. Steps involved in immortalization and tumorigenesis in human B-lymphoblastoid cell lines transformed by Epstein-Barr virus. *Cancer Res.* 2004; 64(10):3361-3364.

[188] Roughan JE, Torgbor C, Thorley-Lawson DA. Germinal center B cells latently infected with Epstein-Barr virus proliferate extensively but do not increase in number. *J. Virol.* 2010; 84(2):1158-1168.

[189] Counter CM, Botelho FM, Wang P, Harley CB, Bacchetti S. Stabilization of short telomeres and telomerase activity accompany immortalization of Epstein-Barr virus-transformed human B lymphocytes. *J. Virol.* 1994; 68(5):3410-3414.

[190] Satoh M, Yasuda T, Higaki T, Goto M, Tanuma S, Ide T, Furuichi Y, Sugimoto M. Innate apoptosis of human B lymphoblasts transformed by Epstein-Barr virus: modulation by cellular immortalization and senescence. *Cell Struct. Funct.* 2003; 28(1):61-70.

[191] Morin GB. The human telomere terminal transferase enzyme is a ribonucleoprotein that synthesizes TTAGGG repeats. *Cell* 1989; 59(3):521-529.

[192] Sugimoto M, Ide T, Goto M, Furuichi Y. Reconsideration of senescence, immortalization and telomere maintenance of Epstein-Barr virus-transformed human B-lymphoblastoid cell lines. *Mech. Ageing. Dev.* 1999; 107(1):51-60.

[193] Sugimoto M, Furuichi Y, Ide T, Goto M. Incorrect us of "immortalization" for B-lymphoblastoid cell lines transformed by Epstein-Barr virus. *J. Virol.* 1999; 73(11):9690-9691.

[194] Takahashi T, Kawabe T, Okazaki Y, Itoh C, Noda K, Tajima M, Satoh M, Goto M, Mitsui Y, Tahara H, Ide T, Furuichi Y, Sugimoto M. In vitro establishment of tumorigenic human B-lymphoblastoid cell lines transformed by Epstein-Barr virus. *DNA Cell Biol.* 2003; 22(11):727-735.

[195] Shiratori M, Sakamoto S, Suzuki N, Tokutake Y, Kawabe Y, Enomoto T, Sugimoto M, Goto M, Matsumoto T, Furuichi Y. Detection by epitope-defined monoclonal antibodies of Werner DNA helicases in the nucleoplasm and their upregulation by cell transformation and immortalization. *J. Cell Biol.* 1999; 144(1):1-9.

[196] Okada M, Goto M, Furuichi Y, Sugimoto M. Differential effects of cytotoxic drugs on mortal and immortalized B-lymphoblastoid cell lines from normal and Werner's syndrome patients. *Biol. Pharm. Bull* 1998; 21(3):235-239.

[197] Fraussen J, Vrolix K, Martinez-Martinez P, Losen M, Meulemans E, De Baets MH, Stinissen P, Somers V. A novel method for making human monoclonal antibodies. *J. Autoimmun.* 2010; 35(2):130-134.

[198] Fraussen J, Vrolix K, Martinez-Martinez P, Hupperts R, Van Diepen A, Meulemans E, De Baets M, Stinissen P, Somers V. Antibody-producing Monoclonal B Cell Lines from Multiple Sclerosis Patients Obtained by B Cell Immortalization. *Clinical Immunology* 2009; 131:S129-S130.

[199] Fraussen J, Martinez P, De Baets M, Van Diepen A, Meulemans E, Stinissen P, Somers V. Characterizing autoantibodies in multiple sclerosis by B cell immortalization. *Journal of Neuroimmunology* 2008; 203(2):183-184.

[200] Vrolix K, Fraussen J, Meulemans E, Becker P, Phernambucq M, Somers V, Losen M, De Baets M, Martinez Martinez P. Monoclonal antibody production by immortalization of B cells from the thymus of myasthenia gravis patients. *Journal of Neuroimmunology* 2008; 203(2):258.

INDEX

B

C

D

E

F

G

H

I

K

L

M

T

U

V

W